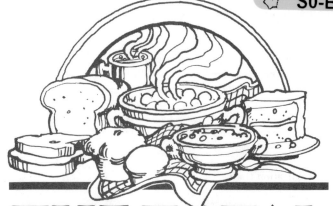

THE TOTAL

fibre

BOOK

A COOKBOOK & NUTRITION GUIDE
FOR HEALTHY LIVING

Margaret Fraser
Associate Food Editor,
CANADIAN LIVING magazine
and
Helen Bishop MacDonald
Nutrition Columnist

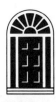

GROSVENOR HOUSE

The publishers wish to express their gratitude to Roussel Canada, Inc., the manufacturer of Fibre Trim, for an education grant which has helped to make possible the publication of this book.

Canadian Cataloguing in Publication Data
Fraser, Margaret.
  The total fibre book

Includes index.
ISBN 0-919959-29-6

1. High-fibre diet. 2. High-fibre diet—
Recipes. I. MacDonald, Helen Bishop, 1939–

II. Title.

RM237.6.F72 1987   641.5'637   C87-093370-1

Published by

Grosvenor House Press Inc.
Suite 375
111 Queen Street East
Toronto, Ontario
M5C 1S2

Éditions Grosvenor Inc.
1456 rue Sherbrooke ouest
Montréal, Québec
H3G 1K4

Printed and bound in Canada
Photography by Fred Bird and Simon Cheung
Food styling by Jennifer McLagan and Claude Arsenault
Cover design by David Sutherland

Book design by Falcom Design and Communications
Illustrated by Penelope Moir
Nutrition Analysis by Sharyn Joliat, Info Access

The publishers wish to thank Villeroy & Boch, Fitz & Floyd and William Smith & Sons Ltd. for supplying china and Kosta Boda for supplying crystal that was used in the colour photographs.

10 9 8 7 6 5 4 3 2 1

An original Grosvenor House Press edition, published for the first time anywhere.

TABLE OF CONTENTS

Fabulous Fibre Recipes 73

INTRODUCTION

Interest in dietary fibre can be traced as far back as 430 B.C. when Hippocrates expressed an interest in the goings-in and comings-out of various food substances and the over-all effect on health.

Well, we've come a long way since then, and fibre has been "in" and "out" in terms of nutritional interest. We are now faced with over-whelming and almost conclusive evidence that fibre, or the lack thereof, can have a definite role in the avoidance or development of particular illnesses and diseases.

Despite the long road travelled, and the general nutrition knowledge accrued along the way, fibre still remains an enigma in the minds of many. What is it? Where do you find it? How much is enough and is there such a thing as too much? Are all fibres created equal and aren't they all just aimed at regularity? Does cooking destroy the fibre content of food? What about chopping and mashing? And just what illnesses are associated with fibre anyway?

This book provides you with the answers to these questions—and any other ones you might have on the subject. More than that, it offers some particular suggestions for increasing your intake of this non-nutrient nutrient.

High-fibre recipes that are both delicious and nutritious are included, along with charts for easy record keeping so that you can get a handle on your current fibre consumption and plot your strategy for future improvement.

This is not to imply that you should be obsessed with fibre—it's one of several important considerations in your daily diet and requires habit formation, like any other good practice.

Acknowledgements

I wish to thank Grosvenor House Press and:
— Regine Farand for her patient and perseverance in
  typing the manuscript.
— Karen Hanley, who organized my material so efficiently.
— Ross Baker, who oversaw the production of the book.
— and my husband and sons for keeping the house going
  while I was writing my material.

Helen Bishop MacDonald
January 1987

Nutrition and Fibre

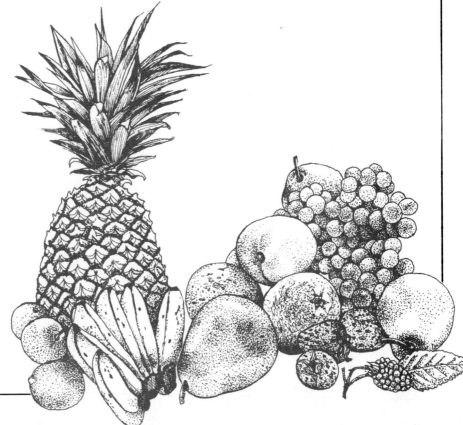

CHAPTER 1

THE VERY FIBRE OF YOUR BEING
Various types of fibre and their functions

*I*t all started in the Garden of Eden. The snake promised Eve wondrous riches and rewards (being as smart as God figured prominently), if she would but eat an apple. And we've been crediting — or discrediting — food ever since.

In the sixth century B.C., Pythagoras took his mind off geometry long enough to advise people to abstain from beans. A couple of centuries later, Hippocrates took a shot at nutrition with the observation that white bread was better than wholemeal since it makes less feces. Well, nobody's perfect. And he did say, "Thy food shall be thy remedy."

Then Galen, right up there with Hippocrates as Greek physicians go, had this to say on the subject: "Let those who refuse to admit the efficacy of food in making men better or more dissolute, more unrestrained or more reserved, bolder or more timid, more barbarous or more civilized, or more given to disputes and fighting, let them on thinking better of it inquire in order to learn from me what they should eat or drink." No shrinking violet, that Galen.

We could go on, but you get the point. Man has always been concerned with his diet and its effect on his well-being and, as a result, various foods and food substances have enjoyed peaks and valleys of popularity.

Fibre is one of those substances that's been in and out like a fiddler's elbow in terms of popularity, and, unfortunately, it has not always been well understood. So to start things off on the right foot, let's begin by asking, "What the heck is fibre anyway?"

Historically, fibre (or roughage if you've been on "Gilligan's Island" for the past ten years) is that dull and inert component of the diet, the stuff that passes undigested from the mouth through the whole digestive system, only to end up intact in the stool.

Benjamin Disraeli was often quoted for having said, "I hate definitions," but since he's not going to read this, I'll give you the definition of fibre according to Health and Welfare Canada's Expert Advisory Committee on Dietary Fibre: "Endogenous components of plant material in the diet which are resistant to digestion by enzymes produced by man. They are predominantly nonstarch polysaccharides and lignin and may include, in addition, associated substances." Seems simple enough, except maybe for the part about "associated substances," more about which later.

Before we can really understand fibre, however, we have to understand the basics about carbohydrates, so bear with me while we talk about such things as hydrated carbon atoms.

Depending on their molecular structure, carbohydrates can be categorized as monosaccharides, disaccharides, or polysaccharides. You don't have to be Einstein to figure out that the monosaccharides are the simplest sugars, and that's because they contain one carbon atom for each group of two hydrogen and one oxygen atoms (that's the water part, as in H_2O). Examples of monosaccharides are glucose and fructose, which you'll recognize from countless labels bearing their names.

Moving right along, we come to the disaccharides, the result of the chemical bonding of two monosaccharides. You'll note that this chemical bonding can occur naturally, in a peach, for example, not just in the labs of chemists who dream up stuff to add to your food. But I digress. When glucose and fructose are the two consenting monosaccharides, we end up with sucrose — table sugar. A union of glucose and galactose gives us lactose, the disaccharide found in milk.

Not satisfied with just disaccharides, nature devised a way of fusing a large number of monosaccharides together, giving birth to the complex carbohydrates known as polysaccharides. The mono's and di's get stuck with the term "simple" sugars or simple carbohydrates, while the poly's are *complex* carbohydrates and get to go to all kinds of athletic events where participants are "loading" up on them.

Most complex carbohydrates, or polysaccharides, are known in the trade (nutrition business, that is) as starches, which comes as a heck of a shock to the carbohydrate fanciers who 10 years ago wouldn't have eaten a starch if it were the last food on earth — remember the potato and the depths to which its reputation sank thanks to Dr. Atkins, et al?

The various carbohydrate-rich foods — our friends, the potato, eggplant or okra, for example — contain various starches, depending on the genes nature handed them. Take amylose — please. This is a starch with hundreds of glucose units marching in a straight line, as it were; whereas another starch, amylo pectin, has these same hundreds of glucose units but with branches sticking out. This is all fascinating stuff, to be sure, but we must get to the ultimate and most abundant polysaccharide on earth — and a major player in the book — cellulose, a component of plant cell walls.

Cellulose and amylose have something in common in that they both consist of glucose units arranged in a straight chain, but after that they're about as much alike as Mother Teresa and the rock star, Madonna.

Because of the way the glucose units are linked together, these two polysaccharides behave chemically and physically in completely different fashions. (I suppose the same rationale could be applied to the behavior of the aforementioned ladies.) The upshot of the whole thing is that cellulose can't be digested by humans, since we don't have the right enzyme to break down the cellulose linkage structure. And herein lies our story.

We've seen now how plants can take simple sugars and turn them into several carbohydrate polymers. Polymers that are complex carbohydrates or polysaccharides, are particular large molecules built up through the linking together of many molecular units.

Getting finally to the nitty-gritty, we may now discuss in all their glory the various forms in which fibre presents itself:

CELLULOSE: A polysaccharide made up of many glucose molecules that are chemically joined; known as a homopolysaccharide, because it contains only glucose.

HEMICELLULOSE: A branched polymer of pentose and hexose sugars. (Remember when I said there were just mono's, di's and polysaccharides? Well, I lied, sort of. Actually, monosaccharides can be classed by the number of carbon atoms they have: Pentoses are five-carbon sugars, and hexoses have six carbons.) Anyway, hemicelluloses contain pentoses and hexoses, the proportions depending on the fruit or vegetable.

LIGNINS: Not even a carbohydrate, lignins are polymers of aromatic alcohols (relax, I'm not getting into that). What they do is encrust the cellulose and hemicellulose during secondary thickening — the older the plant, the more lignin. You've only to bite into an old carrot for an illustration of this.

PECTIN: Straight heteropolysaccharide, pectin is a complex mixture of colloidal polysaccharides. Basically, pectins hold water nicely in an interconnecting network — and that's how we make jelly.

GUMS: Also heteropolysaccharides, gums are water-soluble. Remember this important fact for future discussion. Some gums that you'll recognize from food labels are gum arabic, carob gum and guar gum.

MUCILAGE: Another polysaccharide, this is from seeds and seaweeds and is used in foods as a thickener and stabilizer. Some mucilages show up as bulk laxatives, which you'll also want to remember for later.

From the above descriptions, you'd think that all was neat and tidy in the fibre world, and that measuring it was as easy as weighing a kilo of ground beef. Wrong.

In the first place, there's a fair amount of disagreement in the scientific community about just what substances should merit the term "fibre." Take a quick, second look at all those "fibrous" substances just described, all those celluloses, pectins and lignins. They all behave in somewhat different manners and are broken down during digestion to greater or lesser degrees; in short, what you eat isn't necessarily what you get.

The problem with fibre terminology wasn't born yesterday, either. A German named Einhoff who was wrestling with the concept at the dawn of the 19th century came up with the term "crude fibre". And crude it was. According to Einhoff's theory, after food had been attacked with acid and alkali and otherwise beaten into submission, anything left over got to be called crude fibre. But since hardly anything can withstand this chemical abuse except lignin and cellulose, an awful lot of fibre goes undetected by using this method of analysis.

Well, okay then, why not measure all of the stuff in our diet that resists everything the gastrointestinal tract can throw at it and, to put it as delicately as possible, comes out the other end? That doesn't work well either, because all fibrous substances will suffer to some extent at the hands of intestinal bacteria. Pectin, for example, doesn't stand a chance and not a trace shows up in the feces. We could settle for simply referring to "dietary fibre" — the plant cell wall consisting of cellulose, hemicellulose, pectin, gums and lignin.

Since Einhoff, others have tried to come up with a method that will accurately measure dietary fibre. In the early '70s, a chap called Van Soest developed a "neutral-detergent" method. No, it's not Tide, but it will measure insoluble cellulose, hemicellulose and lignin. The Southgate method is a chemical-extraction procedure that measures hemicelluloses, pectins, gums, lignins, mucilages and polysaccharides. All right, before your eyes glaze over, let's concede that we're probably never going to come up with the ultimate fibre-measurement method.

Given, then, that fibre wears many different faces, let's see if we can't at least get a clear picture of its physical and biochemical properties. Simply put, we know that fibre can be grouped according to four broad functions: 1) water-holding or absorption capacity, which prevents constipation; 2) cation exchange capacity, which simply means that elements such as calcium, phosphorus, magnesium, zinc and iron will bind to various fibre substances (the negative in the fibre story); 3) absorption of organic compounds like bile acids (which lowers cholesterol); and 4) gel formation. Since food contains vast combinations of fibres, the overall effect of any particular food will depend on the content and proportions of fibre present.

THE PHYSIOLOGICAL ACTIONS OF FIBRE

We can state without any fear of contradiction that high-fibre diets increase the weight of the final, residual output. In short, a person on a low-fibre diet can count on excreting roughly 100 grams of stool each day, while his friend, the high-fibre eater, could produce about 400 grams. We're talking nearly a pound! Please note that about 70 per cent of these stools are water, hence the need for more fluid consumption on the part of the guy with the high-fi.

The next well-known fact about fibre is the way it influences the length of time food spends in the digestion process. Fibre certainly prolongs the time food stays in the mouth and stomach, thereby helping you to feel full longer. And it will even delay the entry of food into the small intestine, thereby influencing the rate at which nutrients are absorbed. One of the beneficial things about pectins and gums is that they cause thickening of partially digested matter at about the middle part of the small intestine, causing a bit of a delay in the absorption of glucose (an advantage for diabetics). Now, when fibre-rich food gets to the large intestine, we have truly rapid transit. Movement of fecal matter through the colon is accomplished in roughly half the time for high-fibre eaters versus low-fibre eaters.

We know that certain types of fibre, pectin in particular as well as the fibre of oat bran, will attach to bile acids and cause

a reduction in serum cholesterol levels. We'll discuss the health ramifications of these facts in a later chapter.

Moving right along, we come to another important action of fibre — the way in which some cellulose and most of the hemi-celluloses and pectins are fermented by bacteria in the colon. You may not care for the notion, but fermentation provides energy for the growth of bacteria in the bowel. And, of course, there are gases formed (mostly hydrogen and/or methane) which may be excreted as the passing of wind, or, if absorbed, via the lungs. The level of fermentation will influence the amount of hydrogen in the expired air. This helps explain (much to your relief, I'm sure) the increased amount of gas and possible discomfort immediately following a high-fibre fling, that overdosing on fibre common to recent converts.

Stiff upper lip, now, we're almost finished this part. Another thing I want you to understand is the way in which different types of fibre can influence the type of stool passed. If wheat bran is your choice for extra fibre, then stool weight will be greater, and that extra weight is due strictly to the water-holding capacity of bran. By the way, cooked bran has less water-holding capacity, so more must be consumed to get the same bulking effect. If, on the other hand, extra fruit and vegetables are the source of your increased fibre, weightier stools won't be the result. See the chart on pages 5 - 6 for further functions.

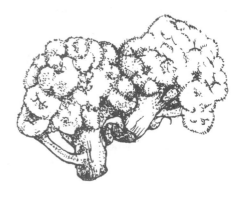

FUNCTIONS AND SOURCES OF FIBRE

FIBRE TYPE	PROBABLE FUNCTIONS	SOURCES
Water Insoluble:		

CELLULOSE	• Aids regularity.
	• May counteract carcinogens in the intestinal tract.
	• Modulates blood-sugar levels.
	• Curbs weight gain.
	• May relieve hemorrhoids and varicose veins.
	• Guards against diverticulosis.
		Apples
		Bran and whole-
		  grain cereals
		Brazil nuts
		Broccoli
		Brussels sprouts
		Cabbage
		Carrots
		Celery
		Green beans
		Lima beans
		Peanuts
		Pears
		Peas
		Rhubarb
		Sweet peppers
		Wax beans
		Whole wheat
		  flour

HEMI-CELLULOSE	• Aids regularity.
	• May counteract carcinogens in the intestinal tract.
	• Modulates blood-sugar levels.
	• Curbs weight gain.
	• May relieve hemorrhoids and varicose veins.
	• Guards against diverticulosis.
		Apples
		Bananas
		Beets
		Bran and whole-
		  grain cereals
		  and breads
		Brussels sprouts
		Eggplant
		Green beans
		Mustard greens
		Radishes
		Sweet corn

LIGNIN	• Lowers cholesterol. • May protect against colon cancer and gallstone formation. • Reduces fermentability of other fibres.	Bran and whole- grain cereals Brazil nuts Cabbage Eggplant Green beans Peaches Peanuts Pears Peas Radishes Strawberries Tomatoes

FIBRE TYPE	PROBABLE FUNCTIONS	GOOD SOURCES
Water Soluble:		
PECTIN	• Lowers cholesterol. • Counters bile acids in the intestinal tract. • May protect against colon cancer and gallstone formation. • Guards against heart disease and diverticulosis. • Promotes growth of bacteria that attack toxins.	Apples Bananas Beets Cabbage Carrots Cauliflower Citrus fruit Dried beans Grapes Green beans Okra Potatoes Strawberries
GUMS/ MUCILAGES	• Lower cholesterol. • Modulate blood-sugar levels. • Promote growth of bacteria that attack toxins.	Dried beans Oat bran Oatmeal Sesame seeds

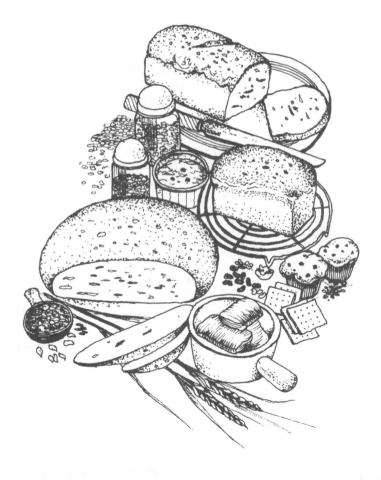

CHAPTER 2

ROUGHING IT UP
How much is enough and where do I get it?

*I*t's been estimated that at the turn of the century the average Canadian consumed roughly 40 grams of dietary fibre daily, with the early '60s seeing consumption levels roughly one-third of that. Current levels of fibre intake show a definite improvement (about 20 grams a day), but the Expert Advisory Committee on Dietary Fibre has recommended that "the adult Canadian population should at least double its intake of dietary fibre."

Human nature being what it is, most people want a number to hang their fibre on. People love numbers: How much should I weigh? How much money should I have in the bank? How many kilometres per litre will this car give me? How many grams of fibre should I eat per day?

Unfortunately, we just don't know enough about the chemical makeup and physiological effects of fibre to be able to pin a number on it. What we do know is that anyone considering an increase in fibre intake shouldn't concentrate on only one source — say, raw bran. Variety is the key with fibre, as it is with any recommendation for a well-balanced diet.

Scientists willing to put a number on fibre intake estimate that 25 to 40 grams of dietary fibre per day is a pretty good ballpark figure. My concern is that we'll develop a generation of fibre-counters similar to the calorie-counters we have today. Better, perhaps, that you learn which foods are a very high source of dietary fibre and which make a poor showing. You can then make routine choices from the

former. An important point to be made here is that while animal products are very poor sources of fibre, foods such as milk, eggs and meat must be appreciated for the great contributions they make of important nutrients. Another thing to bear in mind is that when we're discussing the importance of fibre-rich foods in the diet, we're referring to "routine" eating. It would be a dull world indeed, if one were to suggest that you should never again taste a hot fudge sundae owing to its low-fibre status; sprinkle some nuts on it.

But back to the high-fibre foods — and how much we need. An interesting comparison can be made between some communities in Africa, where estimates put fibre intake at anywhere from 50 to 150 grams per day, and, conversely, the Masai tribes and Eskimos, whose diets contain no food of vegetable origin, and hence minimal fibre. You can see the problem with settling on an ideal number. Suffice it to say that studies indicate improved health for most North Americans where fibre intake is more rather than less. So let's get to the "more."

Beginning with the obvious, it can be said that all foods of vegetable origin, which include grains and cereals, provide fibre. One hundred grams of whole wheat bread (your basic three slices) gives you roughly eight grams of dietary fibre compared with the 2.5 grams you'd get from the same amount of white bread. The point then is that not all plants are created equal — or at least not when it comes to fibre on your dinner plate. It comes as no surprise, I'm sure, that the refining process leaves much of our food wanting in the fibre department. One hundred grams (3-1/2 oz.) of potatoes and most other root vegetables donate between one and three grams of fibre; peel them and you get less.

With any food that's a potentially great source of fibre, the "more or less" rule applies: Leave it alone, you get more, try and make it civilized (i.e., refined), you get less. This is true of old-fashioned oatmeal versus instant; brown rice versus polished; whole-grain flour versus white; fresh fruit versus fruit "drink." About the only food that doesn't suffer from refinement is the bean and members of its family. Even canned beans, other than green and yellow, will give you approximately 20 grams of dietary fibre per 100 grams. Actually, one can hardly say enough good things about this unsung hero of the food world. Since it's rich in fibre, iron and protein, and relatively inexpensive, we'd be hard put to find a negative comment to make about the bean. Well, one does come to mind, for which explanation refer back to the section on bacterial fermentation and gas formation. Nothing's perfect.

The food that hogs all the press for its fibre content is, of course, bran. And there's no denying it, it's a biggie. Just remember, however, that bran (the outer coat of the cereal grain seed) comes from various plants. Not all bran is wheat bran, nor do all brans exhibit the same properties. Most bran that you buy with names like Natural Bran, All-Bran and Bran Flakes are wheat bran. But you can also buy bran products made from corn and oats. They're equally important sources of fibre, but different types of fibre. (Oat bran won't curb constipation, but wheat bran will.)

Pasta has undergone some remarkable changes in recent years, especially where fibre is concerned. Now you can buy not only green (spinach) pasta, orange (carrot) pasta and red (tomato) pasta, but whole-grain pasta as well. I'm not sure what *mama mia* (or even Marco Polo, who is said to have pastafied the western world with his little trip to China) would think of this development, but there's no denying the heightened fibre content of spaghetti made from whole wheat. Sure, it's a different color and one must allow for a certain adjustment for taste (somewhat nutty, actually), but I think we're looking at a winner. Athletes, real or ersatz, interested in a diet rich in complex carbohydrates can hardly do better than whole-grain pasta. The white stuff, really, is the fibre equivalent of white bread.

Nuts are another marvellous source of fibre, so the next time someone says, "Nuts to you," you may thank them for their concern for your good health. Refinement hasn't done much to strip nuts of their fibre content (peanut butter is as good a source as regular peanuts), but the addition of extra oil, sugar and salt is something we could do without. Some of you may have experienced a bout of constipation after an encounter with a jar of peanuts. This is just one of those interesting little anomalies in the world of nutrition; peanuts are loaded with lignin and can sometimes have that effect.

Fruits and vegetables provide various types of fibre, and, other than peeling them, there's not much we do that reduces their overall fibre content. Sure, cooking and mashing alter the nature of the fibre somewhat, but essentially a canned peach contains as much fibre as its fresh cousin; ditto for mashed turnips versus raw.

Now then, to puts things into perspective, and to satisfy that inherent need we all have for charts, let's have a look at the relative fibre content of the various foods that are apt to pass your lips on any given day.

In the Report of the Expert Advisory Committee on Dietary Fibre, it was noted that the adjectives "good" and "excellent" were used to describe food sources of dietary fibre. In the committee's view, these

Fibre Sources

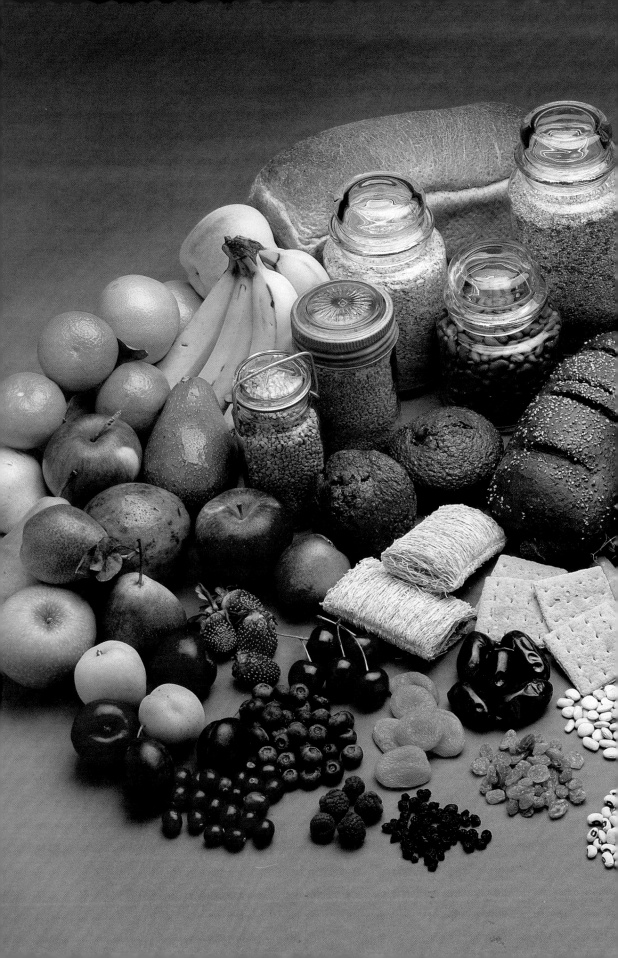

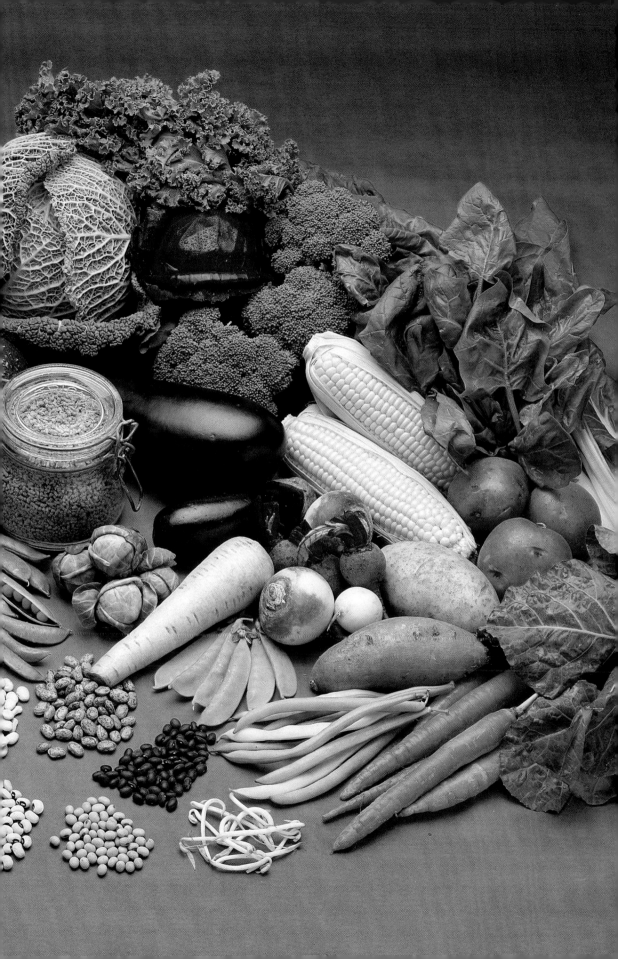

FIBRE SOURCES

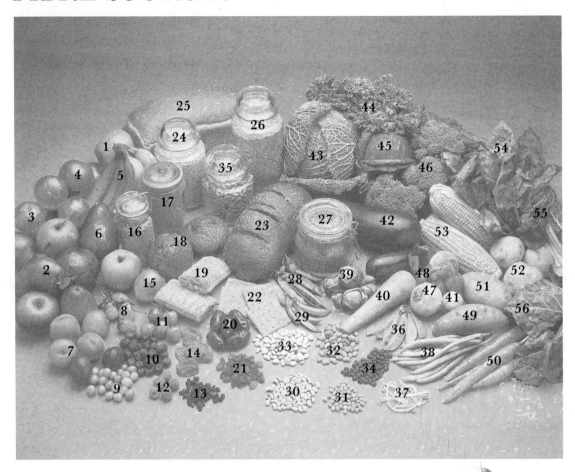

1. apples	20. dates	39. Brussels sprouts
2. pears	21. raisins	40. parsnip
3. clementines	22. graham crackers	41. white turnip
4. oranges	23. rye bread	42. eggplant
5. bananas	24. bran	43. Savoy cabbage
6. avocados	25. whole wheat bread	44. kale
7. plums	26. Red River Cereal	45. red cabbage
8. strawberries	27. all bran germ	46. broccoli
9. cranberries	28. peas	47. turnip
10. blueberries	29. sugar snap peas	48. beets
11. cherries	30. black-eyed beans	49. yam
12. raspberries	31. soy beans	50. carrots
13. currants	32. pinto beans	51. baking potato
14. apricots	33. green lima beans	52. red-skinned potato
15. nectarines	34. black beans	53. corn
16. kasha	35. kidney beans	54. spinach
17. bulgur	36. snow peas	55. Swiss chard
18. bran muffins	37. bean sprouts	56. collards
19. shredded wheat	38. green and yellow beans	

adjectives implied a judgment on the nature of the dietary fibre which could be inappropriate. It was decided that the adjectives used should indicate only the magnitude of the quantities involved.

In keeping with the committee's thinking then, the following is presented:

High Sources

Breads and Cereals
All Bran
Bran Buds
100% Bran

Legumes
Baked beans
Kidney beans
Dried peas and beans cooked

Fruits
Dates (8)
Dried figs (4)
Prunes (5)

Nuts*
Peanuts (100 ml)

Unless indicated all values are based upon 125 ml (1/2 cup) portions.

*High in fat. Don't use too often as a source of fibre.

Moderate Sources

Breads and Cereals
Bran Chex
Bran Flakes
Corn Bran
Cracklin' Bran
Fruit & Fibre
Muffets
Shredded Wheat
Whole Wheat Bread (2 slices)
Cracked Wheat Bread (2 slices)
Rye Bread (2 slices)
Bran Muffins (1 small)
Bulgar (cooked, 75 ml)

Legumes
Lentils

Vegetables
Beets
Broccoli
Brussels Sprouts
Cabbage
Carrots
Corn
Parsnips
Peas (green)
Spinach
Sweet potatoes
Turnips

Fruits
Apricots, dried (10 halves)
Apples (1 fruit)
Avocado* (1 fruit)
Banana (1 fruit)
Blueberries
Cantaloupe (1/2 fruit)
Gooseberries
Mangoes (1 fruit)
Nectarines (1 fruit)
Oranges (1 fruit)
Pear, raw (1 fruit)
Raisins (40 mL)
Rhubarb, cooked
Raspberries
Strawberries

Nuts*
Almonds, unblanched (15 nuts)
Brazilnuts, unblanched, (5)
Walnuts (100 mL)
Filberts, unblanched (100 mL)
Peanut Butter (30 mL)

A few words are probably in order about some of your favorite foods, considered by most as high fibre, that didn't make the list.

Lettuce comes quickly to mind. A cup of lettuce has only 0.8 grams of fibre. You'll recall my mentioning that cooking doesn't reduce the fibre content of food, and lettuce is a perfect case in point. Imagine, if you will, a cooked leaf of lettuce, and what do you have — mush. Because lettuce doesn't have much fibre to begin with, the cooking process really does it in. Celery is usually considered a high-fibre veggie, but a stalk has only 0.7 grams; a small onion, only 1.5. This doesn't mean that these foods don't make important contributions to your nutritional status; they're just not very high in fibre. The same applies to nonfibre foods such as dairy products, fish, meat, chicken and eggs, which provide important protein. Fibre's great, but it's not everything.

To add more fibre to your diet, assuming that your present intake isn't quite up to scratch, a few tips may well be in order:

- The first change should be to whole-grain breads and cereals instead of the refined version. And remember that whole wheat isn't the only game in town. There are some wonderfully interesting breads on the market now and you don't have to go to a specialty bakery to get them. Multi-grain breads, rye and pumpernickel are a few — and the taste is great. The same goes for the new cereals, but don't get carried away in a sea of granola high in hydrogenated fats.

- Brown rice is something that you owe to yourself to try. There are some great new varieties that only take as long to cook as the popular "converted" types and they're not nearly so dull (a euphemism for saying you might have to acquire the taste).

- When snacktime rolls around, reach for things like popcorn, nuts (but not too often, because of their high fat content), dried fruit and seeds. A word of caution about dried fruit: it can wreak havoc on the teeth.

- Think legume more often. I know, it's a strange word, one that doesn't roll off the tongue easily, but there is no end of fabulous dishes you can make with them, as you'll see in the recipe section of this book.

- When making salads, casseroles, puddings or almost anything, toss in some nuts, especially walnuts and almonds, which have fewer calories than a lot of other nuts.

- When buying frozen orange juice, get the kind with extra pulp. With appropriate fruit, leave the peel on. I don't suppose I have to point out that eating banana peel or pineapple rind might be a little extreme.

- Don't automatically toss out perfectly good seeds like those of cucumber and green pepper. The latter make an especially nice addition to salads. So do sesame seeds.

Now to check that you're absorbing what you're reading, you may proceed to complete the following quiz.

MULTIPLE CHOICE

1. The apple that the snake offered Eve was a good source of
    a) lignin   c) wisdom
    b) pectin   d) vitamin C

2. By recommending that people abstain from beans, Pythagoras
    a) denied people an excellent source of vitamin D
    b) diverted attention from his theory on triangles
    c) hoped to corner the Ex-Lax market
    d) reduced people's intake of a high-fibre food

3. Crude fibre is
    a) the material that goes into Joan Rivers' jokes
    b) what's left after food has been boiled in acid and alkali
    c) food that the upper crust won't eat
    d) cellulose and hemicellulose

4. Peanuts may be constipating because
    a) they're very low in fibre
    b) they contain insufficient water
    c) they're very rich in lignin
    d) you always eat them with beer

5. A meal rich in complex carbohydrates would consist of
    a) legumes, cereals and vegetables
    b) dairy products and juices
    c) anything bought in a health food store
    d) milk, eggs and meat

TRUE/FALSE

6. Cooking destroys fibre.
7. Lettuce is an excellent source of fibre.
8. A whole-grain product has significantly more fibre than its refined counterpart.
9. Cornflakes contain practically no fibre.
10. The reason that we humans can't digest cellulose is that we're lacking a particular enzyme.

Answers: 1(b); 2(d); 3(b); 4(c); 5(a); 6(F); 7(F); 8(T); 9(F); 10(T).

CHAPTER 3

A CHIP OFF THE OLD FIBRE BLOCK
Kids are just as fibre-deficient as Grandpa

Just as blanket generalizations are inappropriate in any subject area, such is the case with nutrition. On the topic of fibre, however, we can state with a fair degree of justification that certain segments of the population are more at risk for fibre-deficiency than are others.

Children rank high on the list of potential for inadequate fibre intake and, in fact, it's close to being one of their major dietary problems. Vitamins certainly aren't a problem for the average Canadian kid, since most of them pop supplements from the time they're old enough to watch the "Flintstones". The reason for children's tendency toward fibre inadequacy has not so much to do with their being picky eaters as the type of food they're offered from which to pick: "fun" cereal in the morning with a toy inside (maybe they should eat the toy); juices or fruit drink crystals that offer vitamins but precious little fibre; eggs; milk.

Lunchtime often means every kid's "favorite" meal in a box — macaroni dinner. Again, relatively nutritious, but very low on the fibre scale. With the introduction of whole-grain pasta, we may see an improvement in these offerings. Bread is usually served at lunch, if not as a sandwich then as an accompaniment to the macaroni dinner. If a child is introduced at an early age to whole-grain bread, then that's probably the bread of choice. But woe to the parent who tries to introduce whole wheat bread to a seven-year-old.

Dinner usually consists of some meat, fish or poultry — big on nutrients, zip on fibre.

Accompanying the meat may be some vegetables or a lettuce salad, but the starch source has usually been stripped of any vestige of fibre. The potatoes are peeled, the rice is instant, the noodles are white. Granted, this scenario isn't typical of the diet of every child, but it certainly isn't the exception.

The years pass and all of a sudden we have a teenager (excuse me, adolescent) on our hands. Now we're into "cool" foods, and the food that's "cool" varies from group to group. Two things are certain: The female adolescent is concerned with her weight, and the male adolescent is concerned with his muscles. What's more, both are concerned with the socializing aspect of food, so a pizza or fries after school with the gang takes precedence over broccoli with Mom and Dad. It's not that they don't want to have dinner with the folks, but the girls have had so many calories all day, they can't afford dinner, and the guys don't see cereals, grains and vegetables as the way to "bulk up."

The answer, of course, doesn't lie in nagging about fibre. How about some creative thinking? You could open your very own whole wheat pizza shop; picket McDonald's to serve fries with their skins on and burgers on whole wheat buns. Or, you can make sure that the food in the home, the food to which your teenager is normally exposed, is as high-fibre as possible: whole-grain cookies with raisins, nuts and seeds in them; whole wheat bread, of course; some bran tossed into the casseroles or meat loaf;

fruit for dessert instead of vanilla pudding.

Adults don't get off scot-free either, especially those on a perennial diet, and more especially if their current favorite diet is of the low-carbohydrate ilk, like those of Drs. Atkins, Stillman and company. It seems we have finally emerged from the starch-is-fattening era, but people still can't bring themselves to admitting they eat, even benefit from, starch, preferring instead to refer to it as complex carbohydrates. No matter, the point is that any diet that restricts carbohydrates is a bad diet. In fact, any diet that restricts or overly emphasizes any particular food group is a bad idea.

Now we mosey on into the sunset years and find the worst offenders of all. You can call them elderly, or senior citizens or just plain old, but the fact is that fibre really takes a licking from the geriatric set. Perhaps the story of the old guy with the sore knee helps illustrate the point. When he complained that his right knee was killing him, his doctor observed that he should expect that sort of thing because of his 104 years. The patient was a little puzzled by this, since his left knee was also 104 years old and it wasn't bothering him a bit. This gentleman had successfully eluded the self- fulfilling prophecy, but a lot of his confreres aren't so lucky. And one of the prophecies for which they so readily fall is that once you reach a certain age, say 65, two things happen. You can't handle fibre, and your bowels forget how to do the job for which they were designed. The second item, of course, follows quickly on the heels of the first. Mineral oil and laxatives bring up the rear.

Pity. Because for the most part there's no good reason to think that the colon has gone into retirement just because the rest of you has. And while certain foods may pose a problem for the stomach, or produce extra gas, there's no need to throw out the baby with the bathwater. Sure, eliminate foods that give you a problem, but don't automatically adopt a bland diet just because somebody calls you grandpa.

What you should really focus on, aside from the obvious thing of eating a high-fibre diet, is your fluid intake. Water is probably our most highly underrated "food," and it's particularly important if you're a recent convert and are "branning" everything in sight. A couple of studies have concluded that oftentimes elderly patients in nursing homes who are exhibiting signs of confusion may actually be suffering from dehydration. One of the frequent reasons given for cutting back on fluid intake is the desire to reduce the number of nocturnal visits to the washroom. A valid point, and fluid intake can be restricted after, say, 6 p.m., but during the day make sure that you're tossing back a few — water, that is.

Water, of course, is not the only fluid. Food contains a great deal of liquid, and obviously milk and juices are excellent choices as well. Tea and coffee cause an increase in water loss via the kidneys, so really shouldn't be counted in your fluid intake — which should be six to eight glasses a day — unless they're the decaffeinated variety.

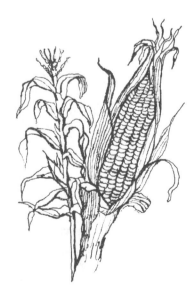

CHAPTER 4

THE VITAMIN BONUS
What else do fibrous foods give you?

One of the neat things about increasing your intake of fibre is that you're not just buying into a beautifully wrapped gift box with nothing inside. As an aside, this is the main problem with the simple sugars — all style (or taste), no substance (or nutrients). With fibrous foods, however, you get a whole raft of hangers-on, nutrient-wise. To be better informed about the contribution to your overall nutritional status, have a look at each of the high-fibre categories and see the wonders that nature has wrought.

FRUITS AND VEGETABLES
When the snake approached Eve, he won her over with the promise of increased knowledge, but I'm sure an equally successful pitch might have been devoted to the nutritional merits of the apple. Don't forget, Eve was a married woman, and women are traditionally in charge of health care for the family. Of course, she was probably already heavily into figs, a fantastic source of fibre, and, if not wearing the leaves, probably made a great casserole out of them as well.

Actually, any fruit or vegetable would have done the trick, since they're such fantastic sources of nutrients, but how do you suppose the Bible would read if the snake's opening line had been "Hey, Eve, have I got a parsnip for you"?

Well, then, aside from various forms of fibre, just what do vegetables and fruits have going for them? They do have some protein, not enough that you could live off

any one of them, but, as exhibited by vegetarians worldwide, enough so that when eaten in combination with themselves or representatives from the bread and cereal group, one can do quite nicely. Their major contribution is vitamins, especially of the B kind, but vitamin A isn't badly done by either, and that's where we'll start.

The type of vitamin A you find in fruit and vegetables isn't, in fact, the real McCoy. Not an imposter, mind you, but what is called a precursor, which will do until the real thing (retinol) comes along. Carotene is what you get from vegetables. In descending order of magnitude, but far-removed from the best source of vitamin A, which is liver (no fibre, but great on flavor), the following list exemplifies some of our most important sources: dandelion greens, cantaloupe, carrots (quelle surprise!), sweet potato, collards, spinach, winter squash (acorn, hubbard, etc., not the summer types like zucchini), beet greens, broccoli, apricots and tomatoes.

All of these are at least in the "moderate" category for fibre, but be careful about overdosing on them. What do you get if you develop a real "thing" for carrots? Orange. That's what tanning pills deliver (a form of carotene), except the ads call it bronze. Orange palms of your hands are part of the deal as well.

The B vitamins, also found in meat, of course, are amply represented in fibrous fruits and vegetables. If you want to avoid beri-beri, which you probably do, then look to things like peas, asparagus, oranges and bananas for a generous serving of thiamin along with your fibre.

Your best bets for riboflavin are liver and milk products, but vegetables and fruits aren't shabby sources, either. Spinach shows up again, followed by asparagus, winter squash, broccoli, soybeans, peas, bananas and oranges. You'll not only be getting plenty of fibre from these foods, but also avoid the dread ariboflavinosis. Not nearly so catchy a name as scurvy or rickets, but just as unpleasant, so make sure your diet isn't short on riboflavin.

Beans figure prominently in the niacin department, but, quite frankly, other vegetables and fruits really don't fare well here at all. Beef and chicken are the best sources, but what they contribute in fibre is zilch. If you're going to eat ethnic, you can't beat a beef and bean burrito when you're trying to ward off pellagra, the disease of niacin deficiency.

And now, a few words about the much-maligned avocado, bound in the pillory because of its fat content. Is there ever a kind word about its content of pantothenic acid, pyridoxine (B_6) or folacin? No. Well, let me say this about the avocado. Surpassed only by liver (wouldn't you know), avocados are just about the best source of the aforesaid vitamins. True, if you're struggling with body fat you don't want to overdo the guacamole (served with your burrito), but as for fibre content and vitamins, it's a real winner.

True confession time now: I have to admit that you could eat fruits and veggies till the cows come home and you'd get not a microgram of vitamin B_{12}, whose sole domain is animal products. Again, nothing's perfect.

But vitamin C! Now we've hit the big time, starting, naturally enough, with citrus fruits. There might also be some fruits and vegetables that will surprise you as rich sources of this vitamin, so beloved by Linus

Pauling. Strawberries, broccoli, cantaloupe, asparagus, potatoes, tomatoes, cabbage, spinach, winter squash and sweet potatoes all provide significant amounts of vitamin C, together with moderate to high supplies of fibre.

Vitamin A referred to earlier is a fat-soluble vitamin; the B's and C are water-soluble, a fact of no minor importance when considering one's daily requirements. Water-solubles tend to be excreted when taken in excess, fat-solubles are stored. Other fat-soluble vitamins to be heard from when considering fibre-rich fruits and vegetables are E and K. (Note that there's no vitamin D, another important fat-soluble nutrient, in fruits and vegetables. If you want it, look to the sun. Which is why Adam and Eve wore only fig leaves and nude beaches have become so popular.)

For vitamin E, you can look to the oils of many vegetables including corn, sunflower, soybean and safflower (has anybody ever actually seen a safflower?). Beans, peas, apples and tomatoes do their bit, as well, but they don't honestly count for much. Wheat germ oil is your best bet.

Vitamin K is found in many foods. Here's where liver, a great source, is beaten hands down — by turnip greens, broccoli and even lettuce. Cabbage and asparagus are no slouches either. And you can count on your friendly intestinal bacteria to produce about half of what you need.

BREADS AND CEREALS

So then, how about those breads and cereals? Not to be outdone by fruits and veggies, these members of the plant family are major contributors of vitamins as well. For brevity's sake, the discussion of their nutrient content will include nuts and seeds also.

Like fruits and vegetables, cereals and grains are sources of incomplete protein, "incomplete" meaning they don't contain the eight essential amino acids — "essential" for human life — in the proper proportions. But combining the various suppliers works wonders. The cereal/bread group is the prime bailiwick of the B vitamins. In fact, you'd be hard put to find a single unit of vitamin A among them, so we'll skip it. D doesn't show up at all; K gets only lip service; and E is mostly dependent on wheat germ oil and oatmeal, if you're trying to find it in the cereal group. You'd have scurvy before you ever found any vitamin C in this group, as early sailors didn't live to tell you. So we'll confine our analysis to vitamin B.

With more than a little reservation, at this point we must say a somewhat kind word about the so-called "junk" cereals. Though it's true they're loaded with sugar and shamefully low in fibre, rendered thus by processing, they have a lot going for them in thiamin, riboflavin and niacin (iron, as well), thanks to enrichment. So someone — read "kid" — addicted to these scary cereals may be denying themselves sufficient fibre, but they're not coming away empty-handed.

Bran Flakes are an excellent source of thiamin, followed by peanuts, oatmeal, wheat germ, brown rice (enriched white rice has it as well), whole wheat and enriched white bread. Bran Flakes show up again for riboflavin, as do peanuts, oatmeal, wheat germ and enriched white bread. The cereal group isn't overly abundant in niacin, but oatmeal figures prominently for biotin, which will help you rest easier, I'm sure.

Brown rice is an important source of pantothenic acid and vitamin B_6, which is also found in wheat germ and whole wheat bread. Folic acid turns up in the likes of wheat germ, whole wheat bread and shredded wheat.

This is but a sampling of the vitamins to be found in foods that are rich in fibre, but the thought may have occurred to you that I haven't mentioned minerals. There's a reason for that, but you'll have to wait for the chapter on problems with excess fibre to find out. I think every nutrition book should have a little mystery in it, don't you?

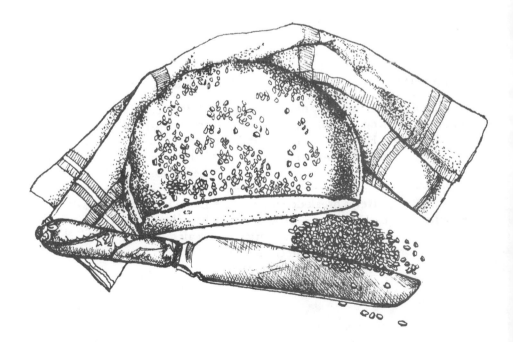

FAT-SOLUBLE VITAMINS

VITAMIN	BENEFITS	FIBROUS SOURCES
Vitamin A (Retinol)	• Helps eyes adjust to dim light. • Keeps skin healthy. • Helps promote growth. • Helps resist infection by keeping linings of mouth, nose, throat and digestive tract healthy.	• Deep yellow fruits and vegetables: carrots, pumpkin, sweet potatoes, winter squash, apricots, cantaloupe, papayas, peaches. • Dark green vegetables: broccoli, spinach, greens.
Vitamin D (Calciferol)	• Helps body use calcium and phosphorus. • Needed for healthy, strong bones and teeth. • Helps keep nervous system and heart working properly.	None.
Vitamin E (Toco-pherols)	• Protects vitamin A and fatty acids from oxidation. • Helps form red blood cells, muscles and other tissues.	• Wheat germ. • Whole-grain cereals and bread. • Green leafy vegetables.
Vitamin K	• Helps form the substances needed for blood clotting.	• Made by bacteria in human intestine. • Green leafy vegetables. • Cabbage. • Cauliflower. • Potatoes.

WATER-SOLUBLE VITAMINS

VITAMIN	BENEFITS	FIBROUS SOURCES
Vitamin B_1 (Thiamin)	• Helps body obtain energy from carbohydrates. • Helps brain, nerves and muscles function.	• Whole-grain and enriched breads and cereals. • Wheat germ. • Legumes.
Vitamin B_2 (Riboflavin)	• Helps break down carbohydrates, proteins and fats to release energy. • Helps resist infection by keeping linings of mouth, nose and digestive tract healthy.	• Dried beans and peas. • Enriched breads and cereals.

WATER-SOLUBLE VITAMINS

VITAMIN	BENEFITS	FIBROUS SOURCES
Niacin	• Helps break down food to provide energy.	• Enriched breads and cereals. • Peanuts, dried peas and beans.
Vitamin B_6 (Pyridoxine)	• Helps the body utilize proteins and fats. • Helps form red blood cells.	• Whole-grain cereals and bread. • Wheat germ. • Oatmeal. • Potatoes. • Green leafy vegetables. • Avocados, bananas. • Nuts.
Vitamin B_{12} (Cobalamins)	• Helps form red blood cells. • Needed for healthy nerves. • Helps form genetic material.	None. (Not available from plant sources.)
Pantothenic acid	• Helps the body utilize proteins, carbohydrates and fats. • Assists in production of hormones.	• Whole-grain cereals and bread. • Nuts. • Dark green vegetables. • Made by bacteria in human intestines.
Biotin	• Helps body make fatty acids. • Helps release energy from carbohydrates.	• Peanuts. • Dark green vegetables. • Made by bacteria in human intestines.
Folic acid	• Helps produce red blood cells. • Helps form genetic material.	• Dark green leafy vegetables. • Dried peas and beans. • Wheat germ.
Vitamin C (Ascorbic acid)	• Works with calcium to build and maintain healthy bones and teeth. • Keeps blood vessels strong. • Protects other vitamins from oxidation. • Helps form collagen. • Helps body fight infection.	• Citrus fruits: oranges, grapefruit, tangerines, lemons. • Strawberries, papayas, cantaloupes. • Broccoli, raw cabbage, mustard and turnip greens, collards.

CHAPTER 5

GOOD FOR ALMOST ANYTHING THAT AILS YOU

Fibre and disease

Next to how to make a million, hardly any area of human activity has generated as much interest lately as fibre intake and its relationship to disease. Constipation, varicose veins, bowel cancer, hemorrhoids, diverticulitis, gallstones, appendicitis, heart disease, diabetes — you name it and someone has fingered it as either being the result of a low-fibre diet or something that can be cured by an increase of fibre. Most of these claims require further study for confirmation, as the Expert Advisory Committee on Dietary Fibre is quick to point out. Still, there appears to be little risk and substantial potential benefit in increasing — as much as doubling — the dietary fibre intake of the average Canadian.

CONSTIPATION

Starting with the most obvious, there's no doubt that in most cases constipation, though not a disease in and of itself, owes its existence to a dearth of fibre in the diet. Emotional stress can exacerbate the situation, giving birth to the familiar admonition, "Don't get your bowels in an uproar." While it's long been known that a fibreless diet leads to constipation, it took Dennis Burkitt and his colleagues to bring the issue to the forefront, and knowledge about fibre and constipation has been growing steadily since their first important treatise on the subject in the early '70s. As you can appreciate by now, it's difficult for me to treat this subject without a touch of bathroom humor, but this is a serious book

and I'll try to dedicate myself to dignity in this section. Constipation is no laughing matter.

It's interesting to note that even bathroom habits are not immune to the vagaries of fad and fashion. In the horse-and-buggy days, it was common wisdom that one had to evacuate oneself on a daily basis, regularity being right up there with godliness and cleanliness. As time passed, that notion was put on the back burner and replaced by the idea that the body knew best and would evacuate itself in its own sweet time; it was silly to be obsessed with having a daily bowel movement. Now the pendulum has swung back as far as a pendulum can swing, to the point that some people are obsessed with the notion of frequent cleansing or purging, feeling that the body is full of poisons and toxins that are sure to do them in if they don't follow some bizarre diet or herbal ritual that behaves as a visceral Draino.

First, let's clear up just exactly what constipation is. Yes, infrequent bowel movements are a manifestation of constipation (which is really a symptom of an underlying condition, not a disease in and of itself) but, on the other hand, the term constipation can also refer to frequent bowel movements consisting of small amounts of very hard and dry stools. Difficulty in passing the stool is another hallmark of constipation, as is pain during a bowel movement or even general abdominal discomfort.

There are any number of medical

conditions that can result in constipation, including hypothyroidism, hyperpara-thyroidism, hypercalcemia, hypokalemia, porphyria, lead intoxication and something called Hirschsprung's disease. You can also be "bound up" by the use of certain "recreational" drugs, antihypertensives, antacids, antihistamines, muscle relaxants, antidepressants, tranquilizers and prolonged use of laxatives. Lack of activity or exercise can be a contributing factor, and there is also a strong connection between constipation and failure to heed the call of Mother Nature.

For the purpose of our discussion, we'll confine our remarks to the role of fibre in preventing or alleviating constipation, when said constipation is, in fact, caused by fibre deficiency. Fibre does two things: it increases the bulk of the stools and decreases transit time through the bowels. Bulk is mostly increased by the way in which fibre absorbs water. It's important to remember that only certain forms of fibre, mainly cellulose and hemicellulose, are water-insoluble and therefore can hold water. (Fibre such as that found in oat bran, for example, does little for you in terms of constipation.) Fibrous material swells up with water and makes big, soft stools — but therein lies the rub. There has to be water available in order for the fibre to swell — hence the earlier reference to the importance of fluid in the diet. You may hold a monopoly on all the bran sales in North America, but if you're lacking in fluid, no go.

Decreased transit time refers to the way, due to extra weight, bulk and softness, fecal matter moves more quickly through the gastrointestinal tract. This is a great boon to regularity and, as we shall see in the discussion on fibre and colon cancer, has other ramifications as well. If you're interested in checking your own transit time, swallow some colored, unpopped popcorn kernels and see when they appear in your stool.

DIVERTICULAR DISEASE
The term diverticular disease refers to a whole range of ailments that can occur in the large intestine. Diverticula (*one* of the little devils is a diverticulum) are outpouchings or balloonings, if you will, (think of a bubble on a bicycle tire) that appear along the length of the colon on the bowel wall. If you possess these outpouchings, you are said to be suffering from diverticulosis, but you usually don't suffer. The suffering comes later, when you develop diverticulitis ("itis" tells you right away that now we're dealing with an inflammation). You can get along just fine with these little balloons, unless inflammation occurs, followed by abscess formation. If you've ever had an abscessed tooth, you'll have a rough idea of the situation. Not so long ago people with any type of diverticular disease were put on low-fibre diets. We've done an about-face on that.

It has now been established that the treatment of choice for diverticulosis or any *uncomplicated* diverticular disease is a high-fibre diet, especially one with lots of wheat bran. Complicated diverticular disease involves such nasty developments as hemorrhaging, when the bowel needs all the rest it can get. Since individual cases vary so widely, blanket recommendations as to the amount of bran that should be consumed are best avoided; you should consult your doctor if you think you suffer from such a disease. However, thrice-daily intake of about two teaspoons of unprocessed bran in conjunction with a general focus on high-fibre foods is usually enough to do the trick, but some diverticula really dig in their heels, and more drastic measures, i.e., more bran, may be required. Then again, some people just can't tolerate bran, and in addition to other high-fibre foods, they may have to look to commercial preparations for help.

Irritable bowel syndrome is one of those puzzling ailments on which medical science doesn't really have a handle. We do know it can affect the entire gastrointestinal tract, and that very likely fibre deficiency is only one of several probable causes. Other physical factors and reaction to stress are usually contributors to the condition, which may or may not respond favorably to bran. "Don't get your bowels in an uproar" has particular relevance to this illness.

CANCER OF THE COLON

I wish I could sit here and write that if you just consume an optimum amount of fibre every day, you'll never get cancer of the colon. I wish I could, but I can't. What I can say is that the whole area is very complicated, both in terms of why fibre may be protective against cancer, and, considering the different types of fibre, which of them does what to whom. Included among the theories on fibre and cancer prevention are:

- It may be the water-holding capacity of fibre, which, by diluting possible carcinogens within the intestines, reduces their cancer-causing potential.
- Maybe fibre changes the bacterial population in the colon, encouraging the growth of "friendly" bacteria that don't form carcinogens from bile salts.
- Perhaps it's the shortened transit time that is protective, since this leaves less time for carcinogenic substances to be in contact with the lining of the intestine.
- It could be that fibre simply traps particular carcinogens and whisks them out of the colon.
- Possibly, fibre interferes with the metabolism of certain bile salts, rendering them unable to produce sterols that form carcinogens.

- Perhaps when bacteria and fibre get together, they produce fatty acids, resulting in greater acidity in the stuff in the colon. This in turn reduces the amount of ammonia, which could be cancer-causing.
- It just might be that fibrous substances are converted into something else that helps prevent cancer.
- None of the above.

Studies on diet and cancer didn't start just yesterday. The first was done in England in 1933 by Stocks and Karns, who found a negative correlation between bread, vegetables and milk and bowel cancer. They didn't go so far as to say those foods prevented cancer, just that those who ate a lot of bread, vegetables and milk seemed to have a smaller risk of getting colon cancer. A study in India in 1968 said pretty much the same thing. Then Burkitt made his famous observations in Africa in 1971, and it really hit the fan — fibre, that is. Since then, many other studies have found a negative correlation between fibre and/or cereal and colon cancer, but some studies have shown no relationship at all.

The studies I am referring to are what are known as epidemiological studies: you look at a large group or community of people, see what's ailing them and try to find a common denominator. So while fibre is one common denominator that can be examined, there are other factors ripe for speculation as well. Take money. Some studies have shown that the more money you make, the greater your chance of developing colon cancer. It probably isn't the money itself that does you in, but something in your lifestyle, or food-style.

A researcher named Michael Hill observed that richer people had a greater concentration of bile acids in their stools. Another fecal bile-acid concentration study compared a group of Finns (who have a relatively low incidence of bowel cancer) with New Yorkers (who have a fairly high incidence). While both groups had nearly the same total amount of bile acid in their feces (don't you find this fascinating?), the Finns produced much weightier stools and so had a lower concentration. One has to observe that there might be bigger differences between Finns and New Yorkers than just the weight of their stools — something along the line of lifestyle.

Another pastime epidemiologists love is to see what happens to groups of people when they move from one place to another. Such studies are done because genetically these groups of people are the same. But by the second generation, each has the food habits of the country in which they live. Favorite groups epidemiologists have picked on are those who moved from Ireland to Boston, or from Japan to Hawaii. Regarding the latter, recent Hawaiians don't have as much stomach cancer as their brothers back home in Japan, but they do have a bit more colon cancer. However, stool weight and transit time are the same for Japanese-Hawaiian fathers and sons, but the sons get more colon cancer.

Then, of course, there's our friend the rat. If there's anything scientists love studying more than large groups of people, it's rats. And with good reason. You can do practically anything (within the bounds of humane treatment) with them. I mean, you can feed them all kinds of different things and see which ones get more tumors at which sites; also, you can study generations of rats in a few years. So as not to bore you to tears with what happened to the two zillion rats that have been studied, the consensus seems to be that high fat enhances, and high fibre reduces, the incidence of colon cancer in rats. The bottom line seems to be that there's good reason to believe that more, rather than less, fibre in your diet has a protective effect against cancer of the colon — but it's not yet

been proven beyond a doubt.

One particular group of fibrous foods must be singled out for special attention: the cabbage family. The first question that pops into my mind has to do with how much colon cancer Irishmen get, but of course they eat their cabbage with corned beef. Anyway, cabbage and its close relatives broccoli, cauliflower, Brussels sprouts and turnip (which isn't exactly a member of the family, but close enough) contain substances called indoles, which also may have something to do with lowered risk of colon cancer.

There's another interesting area regarding fibre and cancer, and that's concerning lignin and its possible role in protecting against breast cancer. In a study published in the journal *Gastroenterology* in 1984, a fellow named Aldercreutz hypothesized that lignin could have a protective effect, owing to the way women who eat lots of lignin-containing foods (whole grains and nuts, primarily) secrete greater amounts of a substance called enterolactone. The particular women studied lived in Finland, and they did indeed consume more lignin and had a significantly lower incidence of breast cancer. The way Aldercreutz tells it, enterolactone may be directly responsible for the protection, or it may knock out estrogen, thought to be connected with cancer, in a manner of speaking. I sure hope I live another hundred years to get to the bottom of this one. In the meantime, pass the nuts.

DIABETES

Diets that are rich in complex carbohydrates and fibre are now routinely prescribed for diabetics. In reality, the diabetic diet is the prudent diet recommended for the public at large by nutrition experts. Coincidentally, it's been shown that cultures who routinely consume a high-fibre diet have a generally lower incidence of diabetes. This is not to say that high fibre "cures" diabetes, or that lack of fibre is the cause of it, but Sherlock Holmes would definitely say there is a link.

Fibres such as guar gum and other mucilaginous compounds — the water-retaining fibres — have been shown to reduce the rate of glucose absorption. One study using a daily dietary supplement of 20 grams of guar gum demonstrated a reduction of the average daily urinary glucose by almost 50 per cent in diabetics. Speculation is that guar gum causes the contents of the gut to become so viscous that absorption of glucose is delayed. Please don't lace up your Adidas and run out looking for guar gum — you're likely to find it only in foods such as icecream and salad dressings, and other stuff on which you shouldn't overdose. And 20 grams of guar gum would be pretty tough to swallow, not being the stuff of which gourmet dinners are made. Other studies have shown pectin to have a similar effect.

In the type of fibre found in oat bran and the bean family (baked beans, kidney beans, garbanzos, etc.), a substance called beta glucans is thought to be responsible for keeping down blood-sugar levels, which may lower insulin requirements after being on such a diet for a length of time. Dr. James Anderson, professor of medicine and clinical nutrition at the University of Kentucky, used a high- carbohydrate, high-fibre diet (called an HCF diet) consisting of 70 per cent carbohydrate, 20 per cent protein and 10 per cent fat in treating diabetics. The insulin requirement for type I (juvenile) diabetics was reduced from 25 to 50 per cent; in type II's (adult onset) by 50 to 100 per cent. And more than 75 per cent of the type II's were able to discontinue their insulin. The basic carbohydrate in the diet was from oat bran and members of the bean family.

Anderson and his colleagues had similar success in improving diabetic control when they used high-fibre diets (70 per cent of the calories as carbohydrate) with whole-grain cereals, leguminous seeds and leafy vegetables. They found that diabetics on less than 20 units of insulin who had been following the standard diabetic diet of 43 per cent carbohydrate were able to maintain control without insulin when they followed a high-carbohydrate, high-fibre diet.

Other studies were able to show that just adding certain fibres to the diet, without upping the carbohydrate to the 70 per cent level, would also enhance control of diabetes. But bear in mind that in these instances a less severe type of diabetes was involved. Diabetes ranges from almost nonexistent, what some may call borderline diabetes, through various degrees of impaired carbohydrate tolerance, to the point of outright, complete insulin dependence. So one doesn't want to jump to conclusions when considering the possible role of increased fibre and/or complex carbohydrates in the treatment of the more severe forms of diabetes.

Dr. David Jenkins, of the Faculty of Medicine at the University of Toronto, is at the forefront of people working to explain just how high-fibre foods affect carbohydrate metabolism. His focus is on determining whether it's fibre itself, or something else in high-fibre foods, that exerts a benefit on the diabetic.

On the other side of the coin, there are researchers who feel that fibre has little to do with the successful management of diabetes, and that it's the weight loss experienced by most people on a high-fibre diet that leads to increased control of their condition. Obviously, more research is needed, and it is ongoing. In the meantime, any diabetic would be advised to work with his physician and dietitian, to routinely consume a diet rich in whole grains, legumes, fruits and vegetables. The usual by-product is a diet that's low in fat, which is bound to be a bonus. This is not to undermine the importance of the meat and dairy groups and the nutrients they contribute when low-fat choices are made.

One of the nutrients present in many high-fibre foods, and absent when they're refined, is a mineral that warrants discussion à propos diabetes. Chromium is that mineral, and since its implication in glucose metabolism in 1959, it has been studied extensively. Not extensively enough to come up with conclusive proof, mind you, but it's an awfully interesting little trace mineral. (Trace minerals get that name because their requirement isn't more than a few milligrams a day.) Though we don't yet have sufficient evidence to state that chromium is an *essential* nutrient in our diet, a provisional allowance has been established at about 50 to 200 micrograms per day.

It has been shown that chromium's function in the body is to help insulin with its job of metabolizing glucose, especially maintaining the rate of glucose removal from blood for uptake into cells. It performs this task in a bound form called glucose tolerance factor (GTF). Low chromium, low GTF, and, presumably, impaired glucose tolerance. Fibre enters the picture as a vehicle for supplying chromium to the diet. Strip away most of the fibre of a food, as in the refining process, and there goes the chromium. Refined wheat flour is a good example. Beef, liver and yeast are also good sources, as is black pepper — but how much pepper can a person consume? It has been shown that the glucose tolerance in severely malnourished children improved significantly after treatment with chromium. Please don't interpret this as a recommendation for chromium supplements — there's no telling what harm you could do

yourself. The chromium story is told just as further evidence of the importance of fibre in the diet.

HEART DISEASE

Epidemiologists have had a field day studying the relationship between low-fibre diets and heart disease. There's very little doubt that cultures in which fibre is lacking in the diet generally have greater problems with heart disease than those where fibre consumption is high. Before we get carried away with this let's point out that where fibre is low, saturated fats are usually high, so there's definitely no clear-cut cause and effect case in these observations. However, there are some pretty good hypotheses.

For openers, we know that people on high-fibre diets usually have low levels of cholesterol in their blood. More than that, specific types of fibre have been shown to bring down serum cholesterol levels when they get out of line. For example, one group of healthy people had their cholesterol levels reduced by 13 per cent after three weeks on a control diet to which 15 grams of pectin were added on a daily basis. Another group had good results when they were given guar gum. You'll recall my mentioning the work of Dr. Anderson with diabetics eating oat bran. Well, guess what, oat bran also brings down cholesterol levels — to the tune of 19 per cent in 85 per cent of Anderson's cases. Talk about serendipity — Anderson actually stumbled on the cholesterol effect during his diabetes research. Again, with oat products and beans, even when the amount of cholesterol in the diet was at 430 milligrams per day, serum cholesterol was brought down an average of 19 per cent in three weeks.

This is pretty exciting stuff, but how does it work? One theory has to do with the way in which some types of fibre can bind with bile salts and bile acids in the intestine, which may be indirectly responsible for the reduction of serum cholesterol levels. In the normal scheme of things, cholesterol is metabolized in the liver to become bile salts, which then take a trip to the gall bladder, and from there to the intestine. Just for efficiency's sake, some of the bile salts may be reabsorbed from the intestine and make the return trip to the liver. At any rate, perhaps fibre keeps the bile salts in the intestine just long enough for bacteria (what would we do without them) to break them down and reschedule their trip into the feces instead. We must note here that not all fibre is hypocholesterolemic, that is, causes a reduction of serum cholesterol. Wheat bran, specifically cellulose, is practically useless for this particular job, thought you'll recall it does have other talents.

Whatever the mechanism, we know that where fibre intake is high, as in certain parts of rural Africa, heart disease is virtually unknown, although it is gradually showing up in African cities. The connection between low fibre and heart disease is certainly not absolute, nor is it universally accepted. It's just another one of the fascinating possibilities linking fibre and health.

OBESITY

If I were to present all of the studies that have been done on fibre and obesity, never mind just on obesity, you would be holding a book the size of the Metropolitan Toronto telephone directory — and just about as interesting to read. I must admit to a personal bias in favor of a relationship between fibre intake and body weight (yes, Virginia, dietitians and nutritionists do have biases like anybody else), so I'll state right off the bat that not all studies support such a relationship.

If one does believe, however, that dietary fibre can have an effect on weight loss, then one must consider the possible mechanism for such an effect. The first thing that

comes to mind might be that fibre promotes satiety, that feeling of fullness one usually equates with Christmas dinner. The argument has been made that if this were the case, we wouldn't be able to say that Chinese food fills you up, but an hour later you want more. But are Chinese dinners necessarily high in fibre? The polished rice isn't; the sweet-and-sour spareribs aren't; nor are the stir-fried beef, the Szechuan noodles or the fortune cookies. In other words, it depends on what you order.

Think about foods that you normally eat that are high in fibre and "stay with you." Baked beans, bran muffins, potatoes. How do you think oatmeal got a reputation for "sticking to your ribs"? If fibrous foods do, in fact, promote a sensation of satiety, it probably has to do with their slower passage through the stomach, and also with the way in which their gradual breakdown results in a gradual release of insulin. As you're probably aware, a quick outpouring of insulin results in a fairly rapid drop in blood sugar, which quickly leads to feelings of hunger.

Another possibility concerns the way in which a diet rich in fibre tends to reduce the intake of foods that are concentrated sources of energy — especially fats. A stomach can only hold so much, and this is true of even the stomach of the most dedicated eater. Unfortunately, most gourmands, or just plain fat people, often focus on low-fibre foods with plenty of rich sauces, followed by desserts inappropriately damned because of their sweetness. It isn't the sweetness that gives them most of their calories, it's the fat. Cherry pie would be a great dessert if it didn't have any crust; of course, then it wouldn't be pie.

It's also true that fibrous foods take longer to eat, and it's been fairly well established that people who eat more slowly are more successful at weight control. You may be familiar with a fad of the early

1900's that convinced people the way to optimum health was through chewing. Horace Fletcher had learned that the British statesman Gladstone had reasoned the human mouth held 32 teeth not by pure chance, but to follow a law of nature that every bite should be chewed 32 times. Fletcher took up where Gladstone left off, and thus was born Fletcherism. Horace got up to about 60 chews per morsel and lost 65 pounds in the process. He also eventually went off the deep end and probably died of malnutrition, but he certainly did establish that you eat less when you chew more.

Some are of the view that fibrous foods enhance weight loss by reducing the efficiency of absorption, so that energy or calories are lost in the stool. They seem to envision a broom sweeping those nasty calories out of the intestine. Personally, I don't put much stock in that theory.

The world of fibre research contains many brilliant and respected investigators doing extremely important work to find a connection between fibre and obesity. In fact, if there were any justice, these men would be household names like Einstein or Frank Sinatra. Among the researchers supporting the notion of increased satiety and reduced caloric intake of a high-fibre diet are K.W. Heaton, D.S. Grimes and C. Gordon — all about as well-known as the fifth Beatle, but nonetheless important contributors to our knowledge of the subject.

It was Heaton's conviction, from a 1978 study, that by inhibiting caloric intake, fibre would naturally reduce weight gain. He compared the feelings of satiety in people eating raw apples and then consuming their caloric equivalent in apple juice, and found the apples scored five times as high in satiety as the juice. In 1980, Heaton studied weight loss in people who ate as much as they wanted of a high-fibre diet, and then repeated the procedure with a low-fibre diet. The caloric intake on the former was found to be almost 500 calories lighter than on the latter. Grimes and Gordon looked at people eating white versus whole wheat bread and had similar results. Satiety seems to play a strong role in determining the likelihood of weight gain or control.

Perhaps, after all, we're puting too much emphasis on weight — or more properly, fat. Didn't the Metropolitan Life Assurance Company increase the acceptable weights for men and women? That they did, but there is nonetheless growing evidence that a wide range of diseases are connected to even relatively mild cases of overfatness. And, unfortunately, in spite of the fitness craze, studies indicate that North Americans are getting fatter. Numerous pieces of research indicate that excess weight is an independent risk factor for high blood pressure, diabetes, gall bladder disease and cancer. Whether or not a high-fibre diet can eliminate some of the fatness remains to be seen, but substituting fibre for fat almost certainly is on the side of prudence.

HEMORRHOIDS

Surely a book on fibre would be derelict in its duty if it avoided the subject of hemorrhoids. A hemorrhoidectomy, the surgical excision of hemorrhoids, is, by all accounts, one of the most disagreeable procedures to which one can be subjected. Even if you don't get to the point of going under the knife, life can be a real pain in the butt for the hemorrhoid sufferer. Avoidance is a terrific idea, and that's where fibre comes in.

As mentioned earlier, it's a well-accepted fact that a minimal fibre intake can lead to constipation. Constipation, naturally, leads to straining at defecation, and this straining will raise intra-abdominal pressure, which most certainly can contribute to the development of hemorrhoids. But can a high-fibre diet cure hemorrhoids? I've personally had several clients, who, on increasing their intake of foods high in cellulose and hemicellulose (basically adding bran and whole wheat bread to their diet plus increased fluid intake), passed softer stools that eliminated straining and definitely improved the situation. One patient particularly stands out in my mind. He admitted to having two hemorrhoids — one was the size of a football, and the other was a real big one! He might have been exaggerating, but he did experience considerable benefit when he increased his fibre intake. One of Dennis Burkitt's findings was that hemorrhoids are almost entirely unknown in rural Africa, where fibre intake is high.

GUIDELINES OF HEALTH GROUPS

We've been talking about the association between a high-fibre diet and the possible prevention of particular illnesses. It would be a good idea, I think, for you to have a look at what various health organizations have to say about fibre within the framework of their diet guidelines. We'll let the Cancer Society speak first.

CANADIAN CANCER SOCIETY DIET GUIDELINES
1. Reduce your total daily fat intake to no more than 30 per cent of total calories.
2. Eat more fibre-containing foods.
3. Have several servings of vegetables and fruits each day.
4. Keep your weight close to ideal.
5. If you drink alcohol, have two or fewer drinks per day.
6. Reduce your consumption of smoked, nitrate-cured and salted foods.

CANADA HEALTH AND WELFARE: NUTRITION RECOMMENDATIONS FOR CANADIANS

In 1977, the Department of Health and Welfare adopted the Nutrition Recommendations for Canadians, derived from the Report of the Committee on Diet and Cardiovascular Disease, 1976. Subsequently, these recommendations were endorsed by provincial and territorial departments of health, professional associations and voluntary agencies.

The guidelines recommend:
1. The consumption of a nutritionally adequate diet, as outlined in Canada's Food Guide.
2. A reduction in calories from fat to 35 per cent of total calories. Include a source of polyunsaturated fatty acid (linoleic acid) in the diet.
3. The consumption of a diet which emphasizes whole-grain products, fruits and vegetables, and minimizes alcohol, salt and refined sugars.
4. The prevention and control of obesity through reducing excess consumption of calories and increasing physical activity. Precautions should be taken that no deficiency of vitamins and minerals occurs when total calories are reduced.

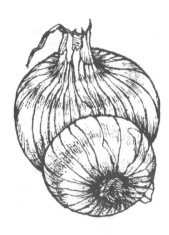

CHAPTER 6

PROCESSING: A TOO-FINE ART
Minerals disappear with hardly a trace

One thing that the 20th century has going for it that other centuries did not (aside from colored television, the Concorde and bubble-gum ice cream) is a wonderful knack for food preservation and storage. As much as some purists might decry the statement, Canadians enjoy a much improved nutritional status in comparison with that of their great-grandparents. Together with improved farm productivity, this is in no small part due to innovations in processing, as well as the preservatives that so many people love to hate. Processing enables us to take foods that are grown in abundance in one area and transport them to another less fortunate region and to enjoy a wide variety of foods all year.

So, there's no doubt about it: Food processing has been a boon to us all, but like most other things in life, there's a hitch. The hitch in this case is that processing not only removes fibre, it removes nutrients as well — particularly trace minerals.

While trace minerals are chemically a whole different ball of wax than vitamins, the two do have a few things in common. The body needs them in only very small amounts; they have a bearing on particular biochemical reactions; and the job that they do is intimately affected by their fellow nutrients.

While it's true that trace minerals are required in very small amounts, it's also true that processing can remove those very small amounts from food. Nutritionists and dietitians are concerned that people may be receiving inadequate amounts of these minerals if their diet consists mainly of highly-processed foods.

When discussing rich sources of a particular nutrient, it's important to consider not only the foods that are the best source of that nutrient, but also whether or not those foods are routinely eaten. So then, with copper we might say that its best sources are not subjected to much refining and let it go at that. Unfortunately, the best sources of copper are liver, oysters and lobster — foods that most of us don't have on a routine basis. The next best sources are whole-grain fibrous foods (wheat and oats) that might be subjected to excessive refinement, including milling and grinding. For this reason, whole-grain products are to be prized over their refined counterparts . . . a little refinement goes a long way. Bran flakes, avocados, baked potatoes, soybeans, bananas, raisins and peanuts — all foods advocated on a high-fibre diet — are good sources of copper.

Zinc is another mineral whose best source, the oyster, isn't the stuff of popular, fast-food restaurants. Again, the milling of grains and cereals will reduce their zinc content. Turkey is a great source of zinc, but in fibrous foods look to lima beans, bran flakes, almonds and peanuts.

Other minerals that are shafted in the refining process include chromium (which we've already discussed — I hope you were paying attention), manganese, molybdenum, vanadium and nickel. (Bet you've been staying awake nights worrying about your vanadium intake, haven't you?) The important point is, I think, that while some refined foods benefit from enrichment, none of them have trace minerals added back during processing, except for iron. This is not to say that refined foods are worthless, or that you're automatically trace-mineral deficient if you've been on a low-fibre diet. It's just another in a long list of reasons why you want to consume more whole-grained, unrefined, high-fibre foods.

It also helps to bear in mind the importance of variety in our diet. The problem is not that we require gargantuan amounts of any nutrient, but rather that we require small amounts of many nutrients — and the surest way to get them is by consuming a wide variety of foods, as long as those foods haven't been overabused.

Remember that it's not just at the hands of the food processor that nutrients can suffer. What you do with your food between its purchase from the grocery store (or even its plucking from your garden) and its appearance on your dinner table will affect its nutrient content. The major indiscretions include indiscriminate peeling and paring, tossing out seeds, chopping or grating too long before serving, soaking vegetables in water before cooking, cutting them too small for cooking, cooking them in too much water (then throwing out the water), and cooking them too long. It takes a pretty tough nutrient to withstand all that.

People love to wring their hands about food losing its nutritional value on the trip up from Florida or Mexico and then being allowed to languish for long periods in the supermarket before purchase. Sure, transportation and long waits in the supermarket can result in some minor nutritional losses, but they're nothing compared to the damage we inflict ourselves. Not only do we often abuse food with inappropriate cooking procedures, many of us also consume insufficient food

for our nutritional well-being (chronic dieters, listen up), or let the fats and refined foods in our diet crowd out those that are rich in fibre and nutrients. Fat and refined carbohydrates are very poor sources of trace elements, the best sources being complex carbohydrates and protein sources such as meat.

A lot of people have also gotten into a stew about food being grown in supposedly nutrient-deficient soil and farmers overfarming the land, then resorting to artificial fertilizers. A few points need to be made here. First, our soil is not nutrient-deficient. There would be a lot more bankrupt farmers if it were. And yes, farmers do use artificial fertilizers and, for reasons of efficiency, thank God that they do.

Historically, it's true that regional nutrient insufficiencies in the soil have caused health problems. You may recall the goiter belts around the Great Lakes, where iodine deficiency was a problem before the days of iodized salt. But the current murmurings that our soil is deficient in selenium and that food processors exacerbate the condition by refining our grains should be put to rest. Again, our soil is not selenium-deficient. It's interesting to note that countries like Finland and New Zealand, where there are marginal levels of selenium in the soil, have benefitted greatly from the importation of Canadian wheat. Most grains aren't a great source of selenium to begin with, so refining them is no big deal in that regard. Your best sources of selenium are foods such as meat, seafoods, eggs and milk.

To know what we'd be facing if we truly had a selenium deficiency, we need only to look at the Keshan province of China. Soil in that area of the country was, unbeknownst to the Chinese at the time, very poor in selenium. Many children were sick and dying with a heart problem called cardiomyopathy. Known as Keshan disease, the illness was found to have a lot in common with a nutritional deficiency that affected animals in the same area. Presto: selenium supplementation to the rescue.

This story may not have a whole lot to do with the importance of fibre in our diet, but it does highlight the need to avoid jumping to conclusions: Canada doesn't have a selenium problem, but there are places in the world that do.

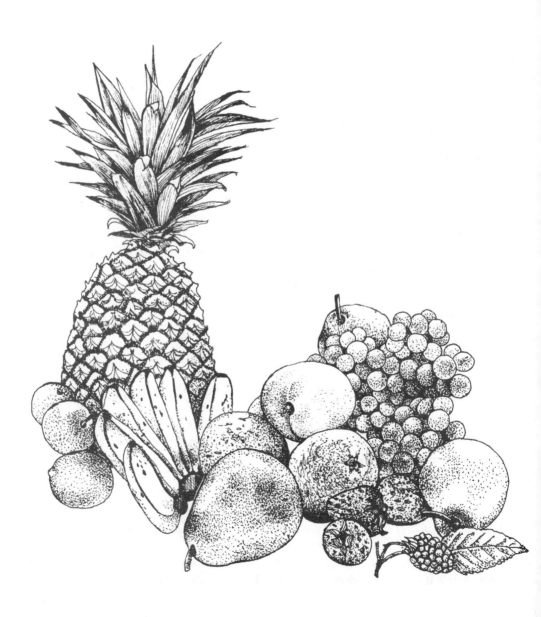

CHAPTER 7

WHEN ENOUGH FIBRE BECOMES TOO MUCH

The continuing case of the disappearing mineral

*U*nfortunately, the old adage, "You can have too much of a good thing," applies to fibre, too. Actually, we're not sure if the too-muchness is due to the fibre itself or to other things that are usually contained in fibrous foods: phytic acid, oxalic acid, or little nasties called goitrogens.

These substances have the capacity to bind with minerals — iron, zinc and iodine, among them — to form an insoluble salt that is excreted by the body. You may be reaping the benefits of fibre on the one hand, but if you're overdosing on excessive fibre on the other, you could be robbing your body of important nutrients at the same time. Note that the operative word is *excessive* — i.e., more than the recommended 25 to 40 grams daily. Remember that the Dietary Fibre Committee noted that most Canadians consume only half the fibre they should.

To begin at the beginning, let's study iron. Iron is present in the diet in two basic forms, heme iron and non-heme iron. The heme form (as in *heme*oglobin) is found in animal products such as liver and red meat; the nonheme form is generally found in plant products, such as whole grains and dark green vegetables. And therein lies the rub, as far as fibre is concerned.

The absorption of heme iron is pretty well dependent on mainly one thing — how badly you need it. If you've been on an iron-deficient diet and one day tuck into a good steak, your body will absorb that iron like a sponge. If, on the other hand, you've been living it up on an iron-clad diet, a lot of the iron in that steak will simply be excreted.

With nonheme iron, it's a whole different story. Being picky about how well it's absorbed, the amount of nonheme iron that is assimilated depends on the whims and vagaries of the food choices of the eater. Take tea and coffee. If you're eating a meal rich in nonheme iron, say, a spinach salad, and with that meal you're enjoying a cup of coffee or tea (even an herbal tea), the amount of iron you get from that meal will be precious little. Nonheme iron isn't well absorbed to begin with, and something in your beverage (maybe the tannic acid, maybe one of the methylxanthines — we're not sure) will further impede absorption.

Since we're discussing a spinach salad, I might as well point out that there's something else in it that will further hamper your iron absorption — and that's the egg. Eggs contain a substance called phosvitin that will undermine iron delivery. In fact, the spinach itself is no great shakes when it comes to delivering iron (Popeye notwithstanding), because of the oxalic acid it contains. Oxalic acid is a substance that binds with minerals (calcium and zinc get bound up, as well as iron), forming an insoluble salt that's excreted by the body.

But hold on, there's good news yet. If your salad has a little meat in it (usually bacon, not the best choice because of the fat), something in that meat, grandly called "meat factor," will enhance the absorption of nonheme iron. The same holds true with the addition of another goodie — tomatoes, or anything rich in vitamin C. This vitamin (ascorbic acid) will greatly improve the amount of iron you get out of a nonheme meal. Wine, by the way, will do the same thing, but you didn't hear it from me.

Knowing, as you do now, the fickleness of iron, let's take a look at what an excessive zeal for fibrous foods can do to this important nutrient. When interest in fibre was rekindled in the '70s, one of the brainstorms that whipped the apostles of fibre into a frenzy was the notion of extending ground beef with soybeans. What a fantastic idea! Talk about killing two birds with one stone; heck, we'd get six or seven. Not only would soyburgers help with the food budget (soybeans being less costly than beef), we'd also cut down on the fat, cholesterol and calorie intake all in one fell swoop — plus increase the fibre intake at the same time. I mean, we're talking Nobel Prize stuff here. Well, when something seems too good to be true, it usually is — and this is.

You remember my saying that the absorption of heme iron is mainly dependent on the body's need; well, I understated the case. A researcher by the name of Walter Mertz showed that when you add soy protein to ground beef, you reduce iron absorption by about half (depending on how much soy you use). (Zinc absorption is affected as well, which we'll get to in a minute.) I'm not sure even Dr. Mertz knows what it is in the soy product that impedes the absorption of iron, but the operative term here is "biological availability," and that is what's being affected by whatever is in the soybean. I'm not saying that one shouldn't consume soy-based products such as tofu to increase our fibre intake or as a source of protein, simply that we might have to bridle our enthusiasm a bit.

Another interesting example of reduced iron absorption concerns the bioavailability of iron in whole grains. You actually stand a better chance of absorbing the iron found in enriched white bread than that in the best unrefined, multigrain product your natural, no-preservative baker can come up with. That has to do with two things: the phytic acid (which behaves like the afore-said oxalic acid) in whole grains, plus the fact that a more readily absorbable form of iron is added to enriched flour.

Am I therefore saying that one should eat white bread instead of whole wheat? No. First, you shouldn't be depending heavily on grains and cereals for your iron anyway (the best source is meat), and the fibre and nutrient content of the whole grain product is a bigger factor in its favor than the iron it contains — unless you never eat meat. (Life's just one big trade-off, isn't it?) Iron enrichment has done great things for cereals as well, Cream of Wheat and baby cereals being two good examples. The bottom line is that if you never eat meat and really overdo it with fibre, your iron status may be seriously compromised. But that has nothing on what will happen to your zinc level.

To tell the zinc story, we'll journey back to Iran circa 1950. At that time, it was noted that there were an awful lot of little Iranian men running around. I mean, *very* little. And they were "running around" because they were sexually immature. The problem was zinc deficiency, and the result was dwarfism coupled with delayed sexual maturity — classic manifestations of the condition. How did such a thing befall these good people?

Again, we go back to the bioavailability of nutrients — especially minerals — and the high-fibre Iranian diet. Not only do whole grains figure prominently in their diet, but also for the most part, their breads are unleavened, as in pita. What's leavening got to do with it? Just that leavening destroys a lot of phytic acid. A diet largely made up of whole grains is low in zinc to start with, since whole grains are high in phytic acid, which binds zinc so that it can't be absorbed. And when there is no leavening of bread to reduce the level of phytic acid, zinc is even further compromised. It's not certain that it was the phytic acid that did them in, or something else in the excessive fibre in their diet, but the fact remains that, despite an abundant supply of zinc in their diet, their bodies just weren't absorbing it.

In an interesting study by Solomons et al, it was shown that if you give a body oysters (the very best source of zinc), most of the zinc will be absorbed. If you give those same oysters with beans, absorption of the zinc is significantly reduced; if you give them with corn, you get no zinc at all. And soya products can have a similarly depressing effect on zinc absorption. Once again, the moral of the story is not that fibre is to be avoided, but that excesses are.

One more mineral to be scrutinized regarding its association with fibre is iodine. It may come as a surprise that centuries ago the Incas, Egyptians and Chinese were treating goiter with iodine-containing substances. Of course they didn't realize it was the iodine that was doing the trick, lacking, as they were, the benefit of dietitians to advise them, but they were right on target. About a hundred years ago, iodine was fingered as the culprit, and goiter was on its way out of business.

Just as is the case with selenium, the soil of some areas of the world has more iodine than it knows what to do with, while in other areas iodine is in short supply. Two factors helped solve the problem: the introduction of iodized salt and the transport system of food delivery, which greatly reduced the likelihood of people being exposed only to foods grown in their own (possibly iodine-deficient) region. This worked well for about 40 years, but now a couple of new wrinkles have appeared.

Some people have become suspicious of anything that big business adds to food, and that includes putting iodine in salt. So they've turned to sea salt for its alleged naturalness and purity. (Can't you just hear the sounds of the sea as you hold a bag of it to your ear?) Wonderfully evocative of the natural life though it may be, sea salt is still just plain old sodium chloride — minus any iodine.

Certain folks (who are often of the anti-iodized salt persuasion) compound the situation by rushing into the cabbage patch. By this I refer to their love affair with the vegetable. Veggies are great, no doubt about it, but certain among them, the cabbage family to be specific, contain substances called goitrogens that compete with iodine for thyroid uptake or foul up the synthesis of thyroid hormone. I want to emphasize that even large amounts of cabbage-family vegetables consumed as part of a well-balanced diet pose no threat. As pointed out earlier, these vegetables have been shown to have a strong association with the prevention of certain types of cancer, and their consumption is to be encouraged. Only those who shun iodized salt and get carried away with all things green and leafy need beware of the effect of an excess of goitrogens that could lead to goiter.

For a real example of goitrogens gone wild, we need only look to certain areas in Africa where a staple in the diet, cassava, is loaded with them; iodized salt isn't an everyday item either. Goiter is common in these regions, but worse than that (goiter probably won't kill you, it will just continue to increase the neck size of your shirts) is the high incidence of cretinism. This condition of stunted growth and mental retardation is the result of prolonged and severe iodine deprivation during fetal development.

With all this talk about mineral deficiencies — and especially if you've missed the point that it's the effect of *excessive* fibre on mineral absorption that we're talking about — you're liable to get the idea that your mineral level is so low you couldn't attract a magnet. When that notion sets in, you could be easy prey for the purveyors of a service called hair analysis. Purporting to analyze your hair for signs of nutrient deficiencies, especially of minerals, these scams are generally just that, if not downright fraudulent. You'll get a printout telling you that your molybdenum is down a bit, and, hey, what about that titanium, and whadda ya know, we just happen to have a dandy little supplement that will fix you right up. Don't you believe it. Granted, there are certain minerals that can be tested for; if Napoleon had had a hair-analysis kit with him on Santa Helena and had clued into the supposed droppings of arsenic in his brandy, the whole course of history might have been altered. But for the average schlemiel like you and me, blood and urine tests are a much more reliable route if, indeed, there is good reason to suspect a deficiency.

More emphasis needs to be placed on the risk of toxicity for individuals who seek to ameliorate a possible or imagined mineral deficiency with varying amounts of supplements. If you decide to try to experiment with supplements — which is strongly discouraged — never, I say NEVER, take more than the RNI (Recommended Nutrient Intake), which you can find in nutrition books in the library or obtain from your doctor or dietitian.

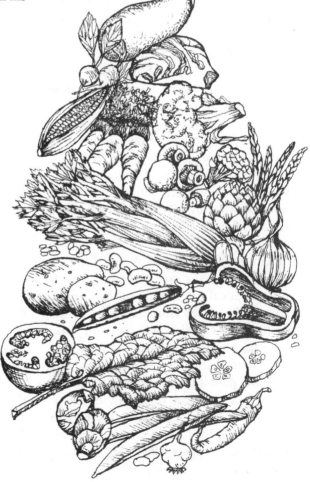

CHAPTER 8

LAXATIVES
Playing loose with unnatural substances

Speaking of the excessive use of anything brings to mind the excessive (on the part of some) use of laxatives. For obscure reasons, there are those who are so preoccupied with the regularity of their bowel habits that they have come to rely on laxatives and cathartics to promote evacuation of the bowel. Since we've just spent a good part of this book discussing the importance of fibre in increasing stool weight and decreasing transit time, you might be wondering just what's wrong with laxatives since they, superficially at least, have the same objective as increased fibre in the diet. The end sort of justifying the means, if you will. The type of laxative that is to be avoided is the "chemical" sort that works by stimulating the large bowel into activity, not those that aid the colon in "bulking up."

Although roughly $13 million dollars are spent annually by Canadians on these chemical "stimulators," you'll seldom find a physician recommending them for any legitimate medical reason. A genuine case of constipation (save one that's so severe it requires medical attention) will fare much better with increased fibre and fluid in the diet, a regular exercise program and good eating and elimination habits.

Don't automatically assume that any lower bowel pain is the result of constipation when in fact it could be symptomatic of appendicitis. The use of laxatives in this situation could have very serious consequences, aggravating an already serious condition.

Chronic abusers of laxatives may also run afoul of the law of electrolytes: Lose a lot of water, lose a lot of minerals — like potassium. Dehydration is a serious problem. Superimposed on that comes a lessening of the large intestine's natural motility. Essentially, one of the main problems with regular laxative use is that, since there are never any formed stools, there's never normal stimulus to the nerve endings in the colon, which in effect say, "Disconnect the phone — nobody ever calls me." Then, of course, the constipation becomes worse — talk about vicious circles.

Aside from the physiological dependence accruing from overuse of laxatives, there's a psychological side to the ledger as well. There are two possibilities here: the case of the person who truly believes that without the use of laxatives a normal bowel movement is impossible, and that of someone with anorexia nervosa or bulimia, who depends on laxatives to rid the body of unwanted calories. Unfortunately, more than just calories are eliminated and the body feels, in the words of Winston Churchill, that this is "something up with which it will not put."

Nutrient loss is bad enough with regular laxatives, but the use of mineral oil really exacerbates the situation, especially as far as the fat-soluble vitamins are concerned. Vitamins A, D, E and K stand nary a chance of absorption when dissolved in mineral oil; they just slide on through. Obviously, the subject of anorexia nervosa is much beyond the scope of this book, but there's one word for using laxatives in the quest of slimness: DON'T.

This is probably as good a time as any to point out that if you've been relying on laxatives, and are ready to seek more natural relief, or simply are set to heed the advice regarding an increased fibre intake, it's best to proceed gradually with additions of bran and such to your regular fare. Remember, much like a newly-made millionaire, your bowels are going to need time to adjust to this new-found wealth. Some bowels may have become quite sensitive, if not downright annoyed, by the goings-on of the past. A sudden onslaught of bran may not be taken kindly. Dean Martin used to joke that he only drank moderately — and he kept a case of Moderately in his dressing room. Take your bran moderately as well.

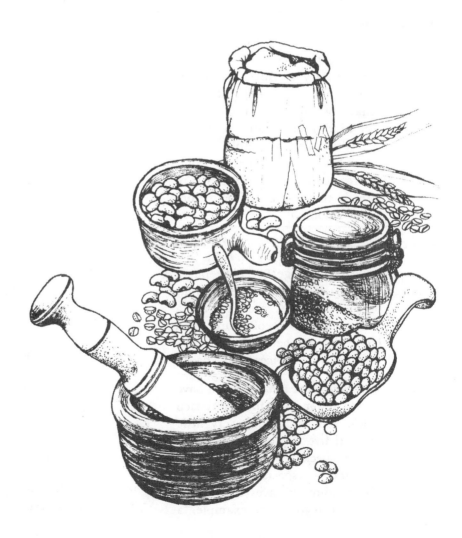

CHAPTER 9

ROUGH AND READY
Putting your fibre where your mouth is

So much for all the talk about fibre; talk's cheap. Let's get down to brass tacks and come up with some concrete plans, *real* habit changes that will bring about a net increase in your fibre intake.

As with a business tycoon planning his next corporate takeover, or a general deciding on military tactics, you have to devise a strategy to help you overcome the obstacle of established habit to achieve your goal. As any general will tell you, you can't determine a course that will get you from here to there until you know precisely where "here" is. In other words, you first have to establish just what are your current eating habits. Therefore:

Step 1. *Record your food intake* for one week by using the Current Fibre Monitor on pages 38-39. Don't try to increase your fibre during this first week — just stick with your usual (possibly crummy) habits. The aim of this game (to use the hip vernacular) is simply to find out where you're coming from; where you're at. Maybe you're already consuming sufficient fibre — but I doubt it.

Step 2. *Compare the foods* you've eaten with the list of fibre-rich foods that appears on page 00. Now put a checkmark beside those of your usual foods that are at least a moderate source of fibre, and circle the number that represents the total fibre choices for the day.

Step 3. *Rate your fibre intake.* If you have chosen fewer than four fibre-rich foods, you are getting very little fibre. If five to eight food choices rate a checkmark, you're in the ballpark — especially if at least two of those choices are in the "high" category, for example, a bran cereal or a serving of legumes. Health and Welfare Canada's Expert Advisory Committee on Dietary Fibre recommended that the average adult should at least double daily intake of fibre. I have no way of knowing if you're "average," but you should be aiming at between 25 to 40 grams of dietary fibre per day.

Step 4. *What are you going to do about it?* Supposing your diet isn't up to scratch, fibrewise, you'll assuredly want to improve things, but remember that changes in habit don't happen overnight. To help you along, we've included Weekly Fibre Calendars on pages 40 to 63. Each day, tick off the foods you eat that are in the "High" and "Moderate" categories.

In order for a food to end up in one of these categories, it had to have been chosen to begin with — and that's where habit-changing comes in. Start by changing your grocery list. Introduce some of the new, high-fibre foods listed on the chart. But also, when wandering down the supermarket aisle, focus on foods that you used to automatically bypass: lentils, brown rice, barley, dried fruits.

When your shopping cart insists on heading toward the cake mix/instant-pudding section, be firm; steer it toward fresh fruit, reminding it of the fibrous benefits. And don't take any sass from it about the high cost of fresh fruits and vegetables. Just let it take a gander at the cost of a frozen cake, never mind the pop and cheezies that other carts are loaded with. The extra pennies for good food are small potatoes compared to the cost of poor health.

Step 5. *Don't be a fanatic* about this stuff. Remember that your *total* fibre intake won't be reflected in the chart; even a glass of orange juice has some fibre, so don't assume that what you mark on the chart is an exact accounting of *all* the fibre you're consuming. Besides, fibre is only one important consideration in your diet — vitamins and minerals count, too. Basically, try to choose one or two High sources and five to seven Moderate choices each day.

For an idea of menu planning around a high-fibre philosophy, the following might prove helpful:

Breakfast	*Lunch*	*Dinner*

PLAN A

Orange juice	2 slices whole wheat bread	3 oz (90 g) lean beef
Oatmeal with 2 tbsp (25 mL) natural bran	Tuna packed in water	Baked potato with skin
	Tomato and zucchini	Spinach
Skim milk	Dried apricots	Whole wheat bread
Banana	Skim milk	Canned peaches
		Skim milk

Calories 1358 **Dietary Fibre** 28.1 gm **Calories from fat** 9.6%
Note: No fat is included for bread and beef used is extremely well trimmed meat.
Recommended Nutrient Intakes for women 19 to 49 years met for all nutrients.*

PLAN B

All-Bran	Pumpernickel bread	Chili with kidney beans
Strawberries	Shrimp	Coleslaw
Skim milk	¼ avocado*	Whole wheat rolls
Whole wheat toast with peanut butter	Alfalfa sprouts	Pineapple
	15 cherries	Oatmeal cookies
	Skim milk	Skim milk

*High in fat, so don't overdo it
Calories 1703 **Dietary Fibre** 36.1 gm **Calories from fat** 28.1%
Recommended Nutrient Intakes for women 19 to 49 years met for all nutrients.*

PLAN C

Scrambled egg with sunflower seeds	Fruit salad	Baked beans
	Cottage cheese	Carrot/raisin salad
Whole-wheat toast	Rye bread	Corn bread
Grapefruit juice	Banana loaf	Apple crisp
	Skim milk	Skim milk

Calories 1588 **Dietary Fibre** 36.1 gm **Calories from fat** 26.0%
Recommended Nutrient Intakes for women 19 to 49 years met for all nutrients with the exception of iron and zinc.*
*"Recommended Nutrient Intakes for Canadians", Health and Welfare Canada, 1983.

CURRENT FIBRE MONITOR

1. Record your food intake, making no effort to change your current diet. The object is to get a reading on the amount of fibre you're consuming *now*.

2. Compare the foods you've eaten with the chart on page 9. Put a check mark beside each item that is at least a "moderate" source of fibre. Circle the number that represents the total fibre choices for the day.

3. Fewer than four choices: You are getting very little fibre. Five to eight: You're in the ballpark, if at least two choices are "high."

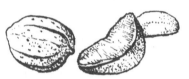

Monday

FOOD AMOUNT FIBRE (✓)

1 2 3 4 5 6 7 8

Thursday

FOOD AMOUNT FIBRE (✓)

1 2 3 4 5 6 7 8

Friday

FOOD AMOUNT FIBRE (✓)

1 2 3 4 5 6 7 8

Tuesday

FOOD	AMOUNT	FIBRE (✓)

1 2 3 4 5 6 7 8

Wednesday

FOOD	AMOUNT	FIBRE (✓)

1 2 3 4 5 6 7 8

Saturday

FOOD	AMOUNT	FIBRE (✓)

1 2 3 4 5 6 7 8

Sunday

FOOD	AMOUNT	FIBRE (✓)

1 2 3 4 5 6 7 8

TOTAL FIBRE PLANNER — *Week One*

High Sources

(4.5 g or more/serving, averaging 5 g/serving)

M T W T F S S **Breads and Cereals**
☐ ☐ ☐ ☐ ☐ ☐ ☐ All Bran
☐ ☐ ☐ ☐ ☐ ☐ ☐ Bran Buds
☐ ☐ ☐ ☐ ☐ ☐ ☐ 100% Bran

M T W T F S S **Legumes**
☐ ☐ ☐ ☐ ☐ ☐ ☐ Baked beans
☐ ☐ ☐ ☐ ☐ ☐ ☐ Kidney beans
☐ ☐ ☐ ☐ ☐ ☐ ☐ Dried peas and beans cooked

M T W T F S S **Fruits**
☐ ☐ ☐ ☐ ☐ ☐ ☐ Dates (8)
☐ ☐ ☐ ☐ ☐ ☐ ☐ Dried figs (4)
☐ ☐ ☐ ☐ ☐ ☐ ☐ Prunes (5)

M T W T F S S **Nuts***
☐ ☐ ☐ ☐ ☐ ☐ ☐ Peanuts (100 ml)

Moderate Sources

(2 to 4.4 g/serving, average 3.5 g/serving)

M T W T F S S **Breads and Cereals**
☐ ☐ ☐ ☐ ☐ ☐ ☐ Bran Chex
☐ ☐ ☐ ☐ ☐ ☐ ☐ Bran Flakes
☐ ☐ ☐ ☐ ☐ ☐ ☐ Corn Bran
☐ ☐ ☐ ☐ ☐ ☐ ☐ Cracklin' Bran
☐ ☐ ☐ ☐ ☐ ☐ ☐ Fruit & Fibre
☐ ☐ ☐ ☐ ☐ ☐ ☐ Muffets
☐ ☐ ☐ ☐ ☐ ☐ ☐ Shredded Wheat
☐ ☐ ☐ ☐ ☐ ☐ ☐ Whole Wheat Bread (2 slices)
☐ ☐ ☐ ☐ ☐ ☐ ☐ Cracked Wheat Bread (2 slices)
☐ ☐ ☐ ☐ ☐ ☐ ☐ Rye Bread (2 slices)
☐ ☐ ☐ ☐ ☐ ☐ ☐ Bran Muffins (1 small)
☐ ☐ ☐ ☐ ☐ ☐ ☐ Bulgar (cooked, 75 ml)

M T W T F S S **Legumes**
☐ ☐ ☐ ☐ ☐ ☐ ☐ Lentils

Unless indicated all values are based upon 125 ml (½ cup) portions.

*High in fat. Don't use too often as a source of fibre.

DAILY RECORD

	Monday	Tuesday	Wednesday
High	☐ ☐ ☐ ☐	**H** ☐ ☐ ☐ ☐	**H** ☐ ☐ ☐ ☐
Moderate	☐ ☐ ☐ ☐ ☐ ☐	**M** ☐ ☐ ☐ ☐ ☐ ☐ ☐	**M** ☐ ☐ ☐ ☐ ☐ ☐ ☐
Totals (approx.)	————————	————————	————————
High	__ servings × 5 = __ g	__ servings × 5 = __ g	__ servings × 5 = __ g
Moderate	__ servings × 3.5 = __ g	__ servings × 3.5 = __ g	__ servings × 3.5 = __ g

(2 to 4.4 g/serving, average 3.5 g/serving)

M T W T F S S	Vegetables
☐☐☐☐☐☐☐	Beets
☐☐☐☐☐☐☐	Broccoli
☐☐☐☐☐☐☐	Brussels Sprouts
☐☐☐☐☐☐☐	Cabbage
☐☐☐☐☐☐☐	Carrots
☐☐☐☐☐☐☐	Corn
☐☐☐☐☐☐☐	Parsnips
☐☐☐☐☐☐☐	Peas (green)
☐☐☐☐☐☐☐	Spinach
☐☐☐☐☐☐☐	Sweet potatoes
☐☐☐☐☐☐☐	Turnips

(2 to 4.4 g/serving, average 3.5 g/serving)

M T W T F S S	Fruits
☐☐☐☐☐☐☐	Apricots, dried (10 halves)
☐☐☐☐☐☐☐	Apples (1 fruit)
☐☐☐☐☐☐☐	Avocado* (1 fruit)
☐☐☐☐☐☐☐	Banana (1 fruit)
☐☐☐☐☐☐☐	Blueberries
☐☐☐☐☐☐☐	Cantaloupe (½ fruit)
☐☐☐☐☐☐☐	Gooseberries
☐☐☐☐☐☐☐	Mangoes (1 fruit)
☐☐☐☐☐☐☐	Nectarines (1 fruit)
☐☐☐☐☐☐☐	Oranges (1 fruit)
☐☐☐☐☐☐☐	Pear, raw (1 fruit)
☐☐☐☐☐☐☐	Raisins (40 ml)
☐☐☐☐☐☐☐	Rhubarb, cooked
☐☐☐☐☐☐☐	Raspberries
☐☐☐☐☐☐☐	Strawberries

M T W T F S S	Nuts*
☐☐☐☐☐☐☐	Almonds, unblanched (15 nuts)
☐☐☐☐☐☐☐	Brazilnuts, unblanched, (5)
☐☐☐☐☐☐☐	Walnuts (100 ml)
☐☐☐☐☐☐☐	Filberts, unblanched (100 ml)
☐☐☐☐☐☐☐	Peanut Butter (30 ml)

Thursday	Friday	Saturday	Sunday
H ☐☐☐☐	H ☐☐☐☐	H ☐☐☐☐	H ☐☐☐☐
M ☐☐☐☐☐☐☐	M ☐☐☐☐☐☐☐	M ☐☐☐☐☐☐☐	M ☐☐☐☐☐☐☐
___ servings × 5 = ___ g	___ servings × 5 = ___ g	___ servings × 5 = ___ g	___ servings × 5 = ___ g
___ servings × 3.5 = ___ g	___ servings × 3.5 = ___ g	___ servings × 3.5 = ___ g	___ servings × 3.5 = ___ g

TOTAL FIBRE PLANNER — *Week Two*

High Sources

(4.5 g or more/serving, averaging 5 g/serving)

M T W T F S S   *Breads and Cereals*
- ☐☐☐☐☐☐☐ All Bran
- ☐☐☐☐☐☐☐ Bran Buds
- ☐☐☐☐☐☐☐ 100% Bran

M T W T F S S   *Legumes*
- ☐☐☐☐☐☐☐ Baked beans
- ☐☐☐☐☐☐☐ Kidney beans
- ☐☐☐☐☐☐☐ Dried peas and beans cooked

M T W T F S S   *Fruits*
- ☐☐☐☐☐☐☐ Dates (8)
- ☐☐☐☐☐☐☐ Dried figs (4)
- ☐☐☐☐☐☐☐ Prunes (5)

M T W T F S S   *Nuts**
- ☐☐☐☐☐☐☐ Peanuts (100 ml)

Moderate Sources

(2 to 4.4 g/serving, average 3.5 g/serving)

M T W T F S S   *Breads and Cereals*
- ☐☐☐☐☐☐☐ Bran Chex
- ☐☐☐☐☐☐☐ Bran Flakes
- ☐☐☐☐☐☐☐ Corn Bran
- ☐☐☐☐☐☐☐ Cracklin' Bran
- ☐☐☐☐☐☐☐ Fruit & Fibre
- ☐☐☐☐☐☐☐ Muffets
- ☐☐☐☐☐☐☐ Shredded Wheat
- ☐☐☐☐☐☐☐ Whole Wheat Bread (2 slices)
- ☐☐☐☐☐☐☐ Cracked Wheat Bread (2 slices)
- ☐☐☐☐☐☐☐ Rye Bread (2 slices)
- ☐☐☐☐☐☐☐ Bran Muffins (1 small)
- ☐☐☐☐☐☐☐ Bulgar (cooked, 75 ml)

M T W T F S S   *Legumes*
- ☐☐☐☐☐☐☐ Lentils

Unless indicated all values are based upon 125 ml (½ cup) portions.

*High in fat. Don't use too often as a source of fibre.

DAILY RECORD

	Monday	Tuesday	Wednesday
High	☐☐☐☐	**H** ☐☐☐☐	**H** ☐☐☐☐
Moderate	☐☐☐☐☐☐	**M** ☐☐☐☐☐☐☐	**M** ☐☐☐☐☐☐☐
Totals (approx.)	_____	_____	_____
High	__ servings × 5 = __ g	__ servings × 5 = __ g	__ servings × 5 = __ g
Moderate	__ servings × 3.5 = __ g	__ servings × 3.5 = __ g	__ servings × 3.5 = __ g

(2 to 4.4 g/serving, average 3.5 g/serving)

M	T	W	T	F	S	S	*Vegetables*
☐	☐	☐	☐	☐	☐	☐	Beets
☐	☐	☐	☐	☐	☐	☐	Broccoli
☐	☐	☐	☐	☐	☐	☐	Brussels Sprouts
☐	☐	☐	☐	☐	☐	☐	Cabbage
☐	☐	☐	☐	☐	☐	☐	Carrots
☐	☐	☐	☐	☐	☐	☐	Corn
☐	☐	☐	☐	☐	☐	☐	Parsnips
☐	☐	☐	☐	☐	☐	☐	Peas (green)
☐	☐	☐	☐	☐	☐	☐	Spinach
☐	☐	☐	☐	☐	☐	☐	Sweet potatoes
☐	☐	☐	☐	☐	☐	☐	Turnips

(2 to 4.4 g/serving, average 3.5 g/serving)

M	T	W	T	F	S	S	*Fruits*
☐	☐	☐	☐	☐	☐	☐	Apricots, dried (10 halves)
☐	☐	☐	☐	☐	☐	☐	Apples (1 fruit)
☐	☐	☐	☐	☐	☐	☐	Avocado* (1 fruit)
☐	☐	☐	☐	☐	☐	☐	Banana (1 fruit)
☐	☐	☐	☐	☐	☐	☐	Blueberries
☐	☐	☐	☐	☐	☐	☐	Cantaloupe (½ fruit)
☐	☐	☐	☐	☐	☐	☐	Gooseberries
☐	☐	☐	☐	☐	☐	☐	Mangoes (1 fruit)
☐	☐	☐	☐	☐	☐	☐	Nectarines (1 fruit)
☐	☐	☐	☐	☐	☐	☐	Oranges (1 fruit)
☐	☐	☐	☐	☐	☐	☐	Pear, raw (1 fruit)
☐	☐	☐	☐	☐	☐	☐	Raisins (40 ml)
☐	☐	☐	☐	☐	☐	☐	Rhubarb, cooked
☐	☐	☐	☐	☐	☐	☐	Raspberries
☐	☐	☐	☐	☐	☐	☐	Strawberries

M	T	W	T	F	S	S	*Nuts* *
☐	☐	☐	☐	☐	☐	☐	Almonds, unblanched (15 nuts)
☐	☐	☐	☐	☐	☐	☐	Brazilnuts, unblanched, (5)
☐	☐	☐	☐	☐	☐	☐	Walnuts (100 ml)
☐	☐	☐	☐	☐	☐	☐	Filberts, unblanched (100 ml)
☐	☐	☐	☐	☐	☐	☐	Peanut Butter (30 ml)

Thursday
H ☐ ☐ ☐ ☐
M ☐ ☐ ☐ ☐ ☐ ☐ ☐

_____
__ servings × 5 = __ g
__ servings × 3.5 = __ g

Friday
H ☐ ☐ ☐ ☐
M ☐ ☐ ☐ ☐ ☐ ☐ ☐

_____
__ servings × 5 = __ g
__ servings × 3.5 = __ g

Saturday
H ☐ ☐ ☐ ☐
M ☐ ☐ ☐ ☐ ☐ ☐ ☐

_____
__ servings × 5 = __ g
__ servings × 3.5 = __ g

Sunday
H ☐ ☐ ☐ ☐
M ☐ ☐ ☐ ☐ ☐ ☐ ☐

_____
__ servings × 5 = __ g
__ servings × 3.5 = __ g

TOTAL FIBRE PLANNER — *Week Three*

High Sources

(4.5 g or more/serving, averaging 5 g/serving)

M T W T F S S	Breads and Cereals
□□□□□□□	All Bran
□□□□□□□	Bran Buds
□□□□□□□	100% Bran

M T W T F S S	Legumes
□□□□□□□	Baked beans
□□□□□□□	Kidney beans
□□□□□□□	Dried peas and beans cooked

M T W T F S S	Fruits
□□□□□□□	Dates (8)
□□□□□□□	Dried figs (4)
□□□□□□□	Prunes (5)

M T W T F S S	Nuts*
□□□□□□□	Peanuts (100 ml)

Moderate Sources

(2 to 4.4 g/serving, average 3.5 g/serving)

M T W T F S S	Breads and Cereals
□□□□□□□	Bran Chex
□□□□□□□	Bran Flakes
□□□□□□□	Corn Bran
□□□□□□□	Cracklin' Bran
□□□□□□□	Fruit & Fibre
□□□□□□□	Muffets
□□□□□□□	Shredded Wheat
□□□□□□□	Whole Wheat Bread (2 slices)
□□□□□□□	Cracked Wheat Bread (2 slices)
□□□□□□□	Rye Bread (2 slices)
□□□□□□□	Bran Muffins (1 small)
□□□□□□□	Bulgar (cooked, 75 ml)

M T W T F S S	Legumes
□□□□□□□	Lentils

Unless indicated all values are based upon 125 ml (½ cup) portions.

*High in fat. Don't use too often as a source of fibre.

DAILY RECORD

	Monday	Tuesday	Wednesday
High	□□□□	H □□□□	H □□□□
Moderate	□□□□□□□	M □□□□□□□	M □□□□□□□
Totals (approx.)	_____	_____	_____
High	__ servings × 5 = __ g	__ servings × 5 = __ g	__ servings × 5 = __ g
Moderate	__ servings × 3.5 = __ g	__ servings × 3.5 = __ g	__ servings × 3.5 = __ g

(2 to 4.4 g/serving, average 3.5 g/serving)

M T W T F S S	Vegetables
☐☐☐☐☐☐☐	Beets
☐☐☐☐☐☐☐	Broccoli
☐☐☐☐☐☐☐	Brussels Sprouts
☐☐☐☐☐☐☐	Cabbage
☐☐☐☐☐☐☐	Carrots
☐☐☐☐☐☐☐	Corn
☐☐☐☐☐☐☐	Parsnips
☐☐☐☐☐☐☐	Peas (green)
☐☐☐☐☐☐☐	Spinach
☐☐☐☐☐☐☐	Sweet potatoes
☐☐☐☐☐☐☐	Turnips

(2 to 4.4 g/serving, average 3.5 g/serving)

M T W T F S S	Fruits
☐☐☐☐☐☐☐	Apricots, dried (10 halves)
☐☐☐☐☐☐☐	Apples (1 fruit)
☐☐☐☐☐☐☐	Avocado* (1 fruit)
☐☐☐☐☐☐☐	Banana (1 fruit)
☐☐☐☐☐☐☐	Blueberries
☐☐☐☐☐☐☐	Cantaloupe (½ fruit)
☐☐☐☐☐☐☐	Gooseberries
☐☐☐☐☐☐☐	Mangoes (1 fruit)
☐☐☐☐☐☐☐	Nectarines (1 fruit)
☐☐☐☐☐☐☐	Oranges (1 fruit)
☐☐☐☐☐☐☐	Pear, raw (1 fruit)
☐☐☐☐☐☐☐	Raisins (40 ml)
☐☐☐☐☐☐☐	Rhubarb, cooked
☐☐☐☐☐☐☐	Raspberries
☐☐☐☐☐☐☐	Strawberries

M T W T F S S	Nuts*
☐☐☐☐☐☐☐	Almonds, unblanched (15 nuts)
☐☐☐☐☐☐☐	Brazilnuts, unblanched, (5)
☐☐☐☐☐☐☐	Walnuts (100 ml)
☐☐☐☐☐☐☐	Filberts, unblanched (100 ml)
☐☐☐☐☐☐☐	Peanut Butter (30 ml)

	Thursday	Friday	Saturday	Sunday
H	☐☐☐☐	☐☐☐☐	☐☐☐☐	☐☐☐
M	☐☐☐☐☐☐☐	☐☐☐☐☐☐☐	☐☐☐☐☐☐☐	☐☐☐☐☐☐☐

___ servings × 5 = ___ g   ___ servings × 5 = ___ g   ___ servings × 5 = ___ g   ___ servings × 5 = ___ g

___ servings × 3.5 = ___ g   ___ servings × 3.5 = ___ g   ___ servings × 3.5 = ___ g   ___ servings × 3.5 = ___ g

TOTAL FIBRE PLANNER — *Week Four*

High Sources

(4.5 g or more/serving, averaging 5 g/serving)

M T W T F S S **Breads and Cereals**
☐☐☐☐☐☐☐ All Bran
☐☐☐☐☐☐☐ Bran Buds
☐☐☐☐☐☐☐ 100% Bran

M T W T F S S **Legumes**
☐☐☐☐☐☐☐ Baked beans
☐☐☐☐☐☐☐ Kidney beans
☐☐☐☐☐☐☐ Dried peas and beans cooked

M T W T F S S **Fruits**
☐☐☐☐☐☐☐ Dates (8)
☐☐☐☐☐☐☐ Dried figs (4)
☐☐☐☐☐☐☐ Prunes (5)

M T W T F S S **Nuts***
☐☐☐☐☐☐☐ Peanuts (100 ml)

Moderate Sources

(2 to 4.4 g/serving, average 3.5 g/serving)

M T W T F S S **Breads and Cereals**
☐☐☐☐☐☐☐ Bran Chex
☐☐☐☐☐☐☐ Bran Flakes
☐☐☐☐☐☐☐ Corn Bran
☐☐☐☐☐☐☐ Cracklin' Bran
☐☐☐☐☐☐☐ Fruit & Fibre
☐☐☐☐☐☐☐ Muffets
☐☐☐☐☐☐☐ Shredded Wheat
☐☐☐☐☐☐☐ Whole Wheat Bread (2 slices)
☐☐☐☐☐☐☐ Cracked Wheat Bread
(2 slices)
☐☐☐☐☐☐☐ Rye Bread (2 slices)
☐☐☐☐☐☐☐ Bran Muffins (1 small)
☐☐☐☐☐☐☐ Bulgar (cooked, 75 ml)

M T W T F S S **Legumes**
☐☐☐☐☐☐☐ Lentils

Unless indicated all values are based upon 125 ml (½ cup) portions.

*High in fat. Don't use too often as a source of fibre.

DAILY RECORD

	Monday	Tuesday	Wednesday
High	☐☐☐☐	H ☐☐☐☐	H ☐☐☐☐
Moderate	☐☐☐☐☐☐☐	M ☐☐☐☐☐☐☐	M ☐☐☐☐☐☐☐
Totals (approx.)	———————	———————	———————
High	__ servings × 5 = __ g	__ servings × 5 = __ g	__ servings × 5 = __ g
Moderate	__ servings × 3.5 = __ g	__ servings × 3.5 = __ g	__ servings × 3.5 = __ g

(2 to 4.4 g/serving, average 3.5 g/serving)

M T W T F S S	Vegetables
☐☐☐☐☐☐☐	Beets
☐☐☐☐☐☐☐	Broccoli
☐☐☐☐☐☐☐	Brussels Sprouts
☐☐☐☐☐☐☐	Cabbage
☐☐☐☐☐☐☐	Carrots
☐☐☐☐☐☐☐	Corn
☐☐☐☐☐☐☐	Parsnips
☐☐☐☐☐☐☐	Peas (green)
☐☐☐☐☐☐☐	Spinach
☐☐☐☐☐☐☐	Sweet potatoes
☐☐☐☐☐☐☐	Turnips

(2 to 4.4 g/serving, average 3.5 g/serving)

M T W T F S S	Fruits
☐☐☐☐☐☐☐	Apricots, dried (10 halves)
☐☐☐☐☐☐☐	Apples (1 fruit)
☐☐☐☐☐☐☐	Avocado* (1 fruit)
☐☐☐☐☐☐☐	Banana (1 fruit)
☐☐☐☐☐☐☐	Blueberries
☐☐☐☐☐☐☐	Cantaloupe (½ fruit)
☐☐☐☐☐☐☐	Gooseberries
☐☐☐☐☐☐☐	Mangoes (1 fruit)
☐☐☐☐☐☐☐	Nectarines (1 fruit)
☐☐☐☐☐☐☐	Oranges (1 fruit)
☐☐☐☐☐☐☐	Pear, raw (1 fruit)
☐☐☐☐☐☐☐	Raisins (40 ml)
☐☐☐☐☐☐☐	Rhubarb, cooked
☐☐☐☐☐☐☐	Raspberries
☐☐☐☐☐☐☐	Strawberries

M T W T F S S	Nuts*
☐☐☐☐☐☐☐	Almonds, unblanched (15 nuts)
☐☐☐☐☐☐☐	Brazilnuts, unblanched, (5)
☐☐☐☐☐☐☐	Walnuts (100 ml)
☐☐☐☐☐☐☐	Filberts, unblanched (100 ml)
☐☐☐☐☐☐☐	Peanut Butter (30 ml)

	Thursday		Friday		Saturday		Sunday
H	☐☐☐☐	H	☐☐☐☐	H	☐☐☐☐	H	☐☐☐☐
M	☐☐☐☐☐☐☐	M	☐☐☐☐☐☐☐	M	☐☐☐☐☐☐☐	M	☐☐☐☐☐☐☐

___ servings × 5 = ___ g   ___ servings × 5 = ___ g   ___ servings × 5 = ___ g   ___ servings × 5 = ___ g

___ servings × 3.5 = ___ g   ___ servings × 3.5 = ___ g   ___ servings × 3.5 = ___ g   ___ servings × 3.5 = ___ g

TOTAL FIBRE PLANNER — *Week Five*

High Sources

(4.5 g or more/serving, averaging 5 g/serving)

M T W T F S S **Breads and Cereals**
☐ ☐ ☐ ☐ ☐ ☐ ☐ All Bran
☐ ☐ ☐ ☐ ☐ ☐ ☐ Bran Buds
☐ ☐ ☐ ☐ ☐ ☐ ☐ 100% Bran

M T W T F S S **Legumes**
☐ ☐ ☐ ☐ ☐ ☐ ☐ Baked beans
☐ ☐ ☐ ☐ ☐ ☐ ☐ Kidney beans
☐ ☐ ☐ ☐ ☐ ☐ ☐ Dried peas and beans cooked

M T W T F S S **Fruits**
☐ ☐ ☐ ☐ ☐ ☐ ☐ Dates (8)
☐ ☐ ☐ ☐ ☐ ☐ ☐ Dried figs (4)
☐ ☐ ☐ ☐ ☐ ☐ ☐ Prunes (5)

M T W T F S S **Nuts***
☐ ☐ ☐ ☐ ☐ ☐ ☐ Peanuts (100 ml)

Moderate Sources

(2 to 4.4 g/serving, average 3.5 g/serving)

M T W T F S S **Breads and Cereals**
☐ ☐ ☐ ☐ ☐ ☐ ☐ Bran Chex
☐ ☐ ☐ ☐ ☐ ☐ ☐ Bran Flakes
☐ ☐ ☐ ☐ ☐ ☐ ☐ Corn Bran
☐ ☐ ☐ ☐ ☐ ☐ ☐ Cracklin' Bran
☐ ☐ ☐ ☐ ☐ ☐ ☐ Fruit & Fibre
☐ ☐ ☐ ☐ ☐ ☐ ☐ Muffets
☐ ☐ ☐ ☐ ☐ ☐ ☐ Shredded Wheat
☐ ☐ ☐ ☐ ☐ ☐ ☐ Whole Wheat Bread (2 slices)
☐ ☐ ☐ ☐ ☐ ☐ ☐ Cracked Wheat Bread
(2 slices)
☐ ☐ ☐ ☐ ☐ ☐ ☐ Rye Bread (2 slices)
☐ ☐ ☐ ☐ ☐ ☐ ☐ Bran Muffins (1 small)
☐ ☐ ☐ ☐ ☐ ☐ ☐ Bulgar (cooked, 75 ml)

M T W T F S S **Legumes**
☐ ☐ ☐ ☐ ☐ ☐ ☐ Lentils

Unless indicated all values are based upon 125 ml (½ cup) portions.

*High in fat. Don't use too often as a source of fibre.

DAILY RECORD

	Monday	Tuesday	Wednesday
High	☐ ☐ ☐ ☐	H ☐ ☐ ☐ ☐	H ☐ ☐ ☐ ☐
Moderate	☐ ☐ ☐ ☐ ☐ ☐ ☐	M ☐ ☐ ☐ ☐ ☐ ☐ ☐	M ☐ ☐ ☐ ☐ ☐ ☐ ☐
Totals (approx.)	_____	_____	_____
High	___ servings × 5 = ___ g	___ servings × 5 = ___ g	___ servings × 5 = ___ g
Moderate	___ servings × 3.5 = ___ g	___ servings × 3.5 = ___ g	___ servings × 3.5 = ___ g

(2 to 4.4 g/serving, average 3.5 g/serving)

M T W T F S S	Vegetables
☐☐☐☐☐☐☐	Beets
☐☐☐☐☐☐☐	Broccoli
☐☐☐☐☐☐☐	Brussels Sprouts
☐☐☐☐☐☐☐	Cabbage
☐☐☐☐☐☐☐	Carrots
☐☐☐☐☐☐☐	Corn
☐☐☐☐☐☐☐	Parsnips
☐☐☐☐☐☐☐	Peas (green)
☐☐☐☐☐☐☐	Spinach
☐☐☐☐☐☐☐	Sweet potatoes
☐☐☐☐☐☐☐	Turnips

(2 to 4.4 g/serving, average 3.5 g/serving)

M T W T F S S	Fruits
☐☐☐☐☐☐☐	Apricots, dried (10 halves)
☐☐☐☐☐☐☐	Apples (1 fruit)
☐☐☐☐☐☐☐	Avocado* (1 fruit)
☐☐☐☐☐☐☐	Banana (1 fruit)
☐☐☐☐☐☐☐	Blueberries
☐☐☐☐☐☐☐	Cantaloupe (½ fruit)
☐☐☐☐☐☐☐	Gooseberries
☐☐☐☐☐☐☐	Mangoes (1 fruit)
☐☐☐☐☐☐☐	Nectarines (1 fruit)
☐☐☐☐☐☐☐	Oranges (1 fruit)
☐☐☐☐☐☐☐	Pear, raw (1 fruit)
☐☐☐☐☐☐☐	Raisins (40 ml)
☐☐☐☐☐☐☐	Rhubarb, cooked
☐☐☐☐☐☐☐	Raspberries
☐☐☐☐☐☐☐	Strawberries

M T W T F S S	Nuts*
☐☐☐☐☐☐☐	Almonds, unblanched (15 nuts)
☐☐☐☐☐☐☐	Brazilnuts, unblanched, (5)
☐☐☐☐☐☐☐	Walnuts (100 ml)
☐☐☐☐☐☐☐	Filberts, unblanched (100 ml)
☐☐☐☐☐☐☐	Peanut Butter (30 ml)

Thursday	Friday	Saturday	Sunday
H ☐☐☐☐	H ☐☐☐☐	H ☐☐☐☐	H ☐☐☐☐
M ☐☐☐☐☐☐☐	M ☐☐☐☐☐☐☐	M ☐☐☐☐☐☐☐	M ☐☐☐☐☐☐☐
___ servings × 5 = ___ g	___ servings × 5 = ___ g	___ servings × 5 = ___ g	___ servings × 5 = ___ g
___ servings × 3.5 = ___ g	___ servings × 3.5 = ___ g	___ servings × 3.5 = ___ g	___ servings × 3.5 = ___ g

TOTAL FIBRE PLANNER — *Week Six*

High Sources

(4.5 g or more/serving, averaging 5 g/serving)

M T W T F S S **Breads and Cereals**
☐☐☐☐☐☐☐ All Bran
☐☐☐☐☐☐☐ Bran Buds
☐☐☐☐☐☐☐ 100% Bran

M T W T F S S **Legumes**
☐☐☐☐☐☐☐ Baked beans
☐☐☐☐☐☐☐ Kidney beans
☐☐☐☐☐☐☐ Dried peas and beans cooked

M T W T F S S **Fruits**
☐☐☐☐☐☐☐ Dates (8)
☐☐☐☐☐☐☐ Dried figs (4)
☐☐☐☐☐☐☐ Prunes (5)

M T W T F S S **Nuts***
☐☐☐☐☐☐☐ Peanuts (100 ml)

Moderate Sources

(2 to 4.4 g/serving, average 3.5 g/serving)

M T W T F S S **Breads and Cereals**
☐☐☐☐☐☐☐ Bran Chex
☐☐☐☐☐☐☐ Bran Flakes
☐☐☐☐☐☐☐ Corn Bran
☐☐☐☐☐☐☐ Cracklin' Bran
☐☐☐☐☐☐☐ Fruit & Fibre
☐☐☐☐☐☐☐ Muffets
☐☐☐☐☐☐☐ Shredded Wheat
☐☐☐☐☐☐☐ Whole Wheat Bread (2 slices)
☐☐☐☐☐☐☐ Cracked Wheat Bread
(2 slices)
☐☐☐☐☐☐☐ Rye Bread (2 slices)
☐☐☐☐☐☐☐ Bran Muffins (1 small)
☐☐☐☐☐☐☐ Bulgar (cooked, 75 ml)

M T W T F S S **Legumes**
☐☐☐☐☐☐☐ Lentils

Unless indicated all values are based upon 125 ml (½ cup) portions.

*High in fat. Don't use too often as a source of fibre.

DAILY RECORD

	Monday	Tuesday	Wednesday
High	☐☐☐☐	H ☐☐☐☐	H ☐☐☐☐
Moderate	☐☐☐☐☐☐☐	M ☐☐☐☐☐☐☐	M ☐☐☐☐☐☐☐
Totals (approx.)	_____	_____	_____
High	__ servings × 5 = __ g	__ servings × 5 = __ g	__ servings × 5 = __ g
Moderate	__ servings × 3.5 = __ g	__ servings × 3.5 = __ g	__ servings × 3.5 = __ g

(2 to 4.4 g/serving, average 3.5 g/serving)

M T W T F S S	Vegetables
□□□□□□□	Beets
□□□□□□□	Broccoli
□□□□□□□	Brussels Sprouts
□□□□□□□	Cabbage
□□□□□□□	Carrots
□□□□□□□	Corn
□□□□□□□	Parsnips
□□□□□□□	Peas (green)
□□□□□□□	Spinach
□□□□□□□	Sweet potatoes
□□□□□□□	Turnips

(2 to 4.4 g/serving, average 3.5 g/serving)

M T W T F S S	Fruits
□□□□□□□	Apricots, dried (10 halves)
□□□□□□□	Apples (1 fruit)
□□□□□□□	Avocado* (1 fruit)
□□□□□□□	Banana (1 fruit)
□□□□□□□	Blueberries
□□□□□□□	Cantaloupe (½ fruit)
□□□□□□□	Gooseberries
□□□□□□□	Mangoes (1 fruit)
□□□□□□□	Nectarines (1 fruit)
□□□□□□□	Oranges (1 fruit)
□□□□□□□	Pear, raw (1 fruit)
□□□□□□□	Raisins (40 ml)
□□□□□□□	Rhubarb, cooked
□□□□□□□	Raspberries
□□□□□□□	Strawberries

M T W T F S S	Nuts*
□□□□□□□	Almonds, unblanched (15 nuts)
□□□□□□□	Brazilnuts, unblanched, (5)
□□□□□□□	Walnuts (100 ml)
□□□□□□□	Filberts, unblanched (100 ml)
□□□□□□□	Peanut Butter (30 ml)

Thursday	Friday	Saturday	Sunday
H □□□□	H □□□□	H □□□□	H □□□□
M □□□□□□□	M □□□□□□□	M □□□□□□□	M □□□□□□□
___ servings × 5 = ___ g	___ servings × 5 = ___ g	___ servings × 5 = ___ g	___ servings × 5 = ___ g
___ servings × 3.5 = ___ g	___ servings × 3.5 = ___ g	___ servings × 3.5 = ___ g	___ servings × 3.5 = ___ g

TOTAL FIBRE PLANNER — *Week Seven*

High Sources

(4.5 g or more/serving, averaging 5 g/serving)

M T W T F S S **Breads and Cereals**
☐ ☐ ☐ ☐ ☐ ☐ ☐ All Bran
☐ ☐ ☐ ☐ ☐ ☐ ☐ Bran Buds
☐ ☐ ☐ ☐ ☐ ☐ ☐ 100% Bran

M T W T F S S **Legumes**
☐ ☐ ☐ ☐ ☐ ☐ ☐ Baked beans
☐ ☐ ☐ ☐ ☐ ☐ ☐ Kidney beans
☐ ☐ ☐ ☐ ☐ ☐ ☐ Dried peas and beans cooked

M T W T F S S **Fruits**
☐ ☐ ☐ ☐ ☐ ☐ ☐ Dates (8)
☐ ☐ ☐ ☐ ☐ ☐ ☐ Dried figs (4)
☐ ☐ ☐ ☐ ☐ ☐ ☐ Prunes (5)

M T W T F S S **Nuts** *
☐ ☐ ☐ ☐ ☐ ☐ ☐ Peanuts (100 ml)

Moderate Sources

(2 to 4.4 g/serving, average 3.5 g/serving)

M T W T F S S **Breads and Cereals**
☐ ☐ ☐ ☐ ☐ ☐ ☐ Bran Chex
☐ ☐ ☐ ☐ ☐ ☐ ☐ Bran Flakes
☐ ☐ ☐ ☐ ☐ ☐ ☐ Corn Bran
☐ ☐ ☐ ☐ ☐ ☐ ☐ Cracklin' Bran
☐ ☐ ☐ ☐ ☐ ☐ ☐ Fruit & Fibre
☐ ☐ ☐ ☐ ☐ ☐ ☐ Muffets
☐ ☐ ☐ ☐ ☐ ☐ ☐ Shredded Wheat
☐ ☐ ☐ ☐ ☐ ☐ ☐ Whole Wheat Bread (2 slices)
☐ ☐ ☐ ☐ ☐ ☐ ☐ Cracked Wheat Bread (2 slices)
☐ ☐ ☐ ☐ ☐ ☐ ☐ Rye Bread (2 slices)
☐ ☐ ☐ ☐ ☐ ☐ ☐ Bran Muffins (1 small)
☐ ☐ ☐ ☐ ☐ ☐ ☐ Bulgar (cooked, 75 ml)

M T W T F S S **Legumes**
☐ ☐ ☐ ☐ ☐ ☐ ☐ Lentils

Unless indicated all values are based upon 125 ml (½ cup) portions.

*High in fat. Don't use too often as a source of fibre.

DAILY RECORD

	Monday	Tuesday	Wednesday
High	☐ ☐ ☐ ☐	H ☐ ☐ ☐ ☐	H ☐ ☐ ☐ ☐
Moderate	☐ ☐ ☐ ☐ ☐ ☐ ☐	M ☐ ☐ ☐ ☐ ☐ ☐ ☐	M ☐ ☐ ☐ ☐ ☐ ☐ ☐
Totals (approx.)	————————	————————	————————
High	__ servings × 5 = __ g	__ servings × 5 = __ g	__ servings × 5 = __ g
Moderate	__ servings × 3.5 = __ g	__ servings × 3.5 = __ g	__ servings × 3.5 = __ g

(2 to 4.4 g/serving, average 3.5 g/serving)

M T W T F S S	Vegetables
☐☐☐☐☐☐☐	Beets
☐☐☐☐☐☐☐	Broccoli
☐☐☐☐☐☐☐	Brussels Sprouts
☐☐☐☐☐☐☐	Cabbage
☐☐☐☐☐☐☐	Carrots
☐☐☐☐☐☐☐	Corn
☐☐☐☐☐☐☐	Parsnips
☐☐☐☐☐☐☐	Peas (green)
☐☐☐☐☐☐☐	Spinach
☐☐☐☐☐☐☐	Sweet potatoes
☐☐☐☐☐☐☐	Turnips

(2 to 4.4 g/serving, average 3.5 g/serving)

M T W T F S S	Fruits
☐☐☐☐☐☐☐	Apricots, dried (10 halves)
☐☐☐☐☐☐☐	Apples (1 fruit)
☐☐☐☐☐☐☐	Avocado* (1 fruit)
☐☐☐☐☐☐☐	Banana (1 fruit)
☐☐☐☐☐☐☐	Blueberries
☐☐☐☐☐☐☐	Cantaloupe (½ fruit)
☐☐☐☐☐☐☐	Gooseberries
☐☐☐☐☐☐☐	Mangoes (1 fruit)
☐☐☐☐☐☐☐	Nectarines (1 fruit)
☐☐☐☐☐☐☐	Oranges (1 fruit)
☐☐☐☐☐☐☐	Pear, raw (1 fruit)
☐☐☐☐☐☐☐	Raisins (40 ml)
☐☐☐☐☐☐☐	Rhubarb, cooked
☐☐☐☐☐☐☐	Raspberries
☐☐☐☐☐☐☐	Strawberries

M T W T F S S	Nuts*
☐☐☐☐☐☐☐	Almonds, unblanched (15 nuts)
☐☐☐☐☐☐☐	Brazilnuts, unblanched, (5)
☐☐☐☐☐☐☐	Walnuts (100 ml)
☐☐☐☐☐☐☐	Filberts, unblanched (100 ml)
☐☐☐☐☐☐☐	Peanut Butter (30 ml)

Thursday	Friday	Saturday	Sunday
☐☐☐☐ ☐	H ☐☐☐☐	H ☐☐☐☐	H ☐☐☐☐
☐☐☐☐☐☐☐☐	M ☐☐☐☐☐☐☐☐	M ☐☐☐☐☐☐☐☐	M ☐☐☐☐☐☐☐☐
__ servings × 5 = __ g	__ servings × 5 = __ g	__ servings × 5 = __ g	__ servings × 5 = __ g
__ servings × 3.5 = __ g	__ servings × 3.5 = __ g	__ servings × 3.5 = __ g	__ servings × 3.5 = __ g

TOTAL FIBRE PLANNER — *Week Eight*

High Sources

(4.5 g or more/serving, averaging 5 g/serving)

M T W T F S S **Breads and Cereals**
☐☐☐☐☐☐☐ All Bran
☐☐☐☐☐☐☐ Bran Buds
☐☐☐☐☐☐☐ 100% Bran

M T W T F S S **Legumes**
☐☐☐☐☐☐☐ Baked beans
☐☐☐☐☐☐☐ Kidney beans
☐☐☐☐☐☐☐ Dried peas and beans cooked

M T W T F S S **Fruits**
☐☐☐☐☐☐☐ Dates (8)
☐☐☐☐☐☐☐ Dried figs (4)
☐☐☐☐☐☐☐ Prunes (5)

M T W T F S S **Nuts***
☐☐☐☐☐☐☐ Peanuts (100 ml)

Moderate Sources

(2 to 4.4 g/serving, average 3.5 g/serving)

M T W T F S S **Breads and Cereals**
☐☐☐☐☐☐☐ Bran Chex
☐☐☐☐☐☐☐ Bran Flakes
☐☐☐☐☐☐☐ Corn Bran
☐☐☐☐☐☐☐ Cracklin' Bran
☐☐☐☐☐☐☐ Fruit & Fibre
☐☐☐☐☐☐☐ Muffets
☐☐☐☐☐☐☐ Shredded Wheat
☐☐☐☐☐☐☐ Whole Wheat Bread (2 slices)
☐☐☐☐☐☐☐ Cracked Wheat Bread
        (2 slices)
☐☐☐☐☐☐☐ Rye Bread (2 slices)
☐☐☐☐☐☐☐ Bran Muffins (1 small)
☐☐☐☐☐☐☐ Bulgar (cooked, 75 ml)

M T W T F S S **Legumes**
☐☐☐☐☐☐☐ Lentils

Unless indicated all values are based upon 125 ml (½ cup) portions.

*High in fat. Don't use too often as a source of fibre.

DAILY RECORD

	Monday	Tuesday	Wednesday
High	☐☐☐☐	H ☐☐☐☐	H ☐☐☐☐
Moderate	☐☐☐☐☐☐☐	M ☐☐☐☐☐☐☐	M ☐☐☐☐☐☐☐
Totals (approx.)	_____	_____	_____
High	__ servings × 5 = __ g	__ servings × 5 = __ g	__ servings × 5 = __ g
Moderate	__ servings × 3.5 = __ g	__ servings × 3.5 = __ g	__ servings × 3.5 = __ g

(2 to 4.4 g/serving, average 3.5 g/serving)

M T W T F S S	Vegetables
□□□□□□□	Beets
□□□□□□□	Broccoli
□□□□□□□	Brussels Sprouts
□□□□□□□	Cabbage
□□□□□□□	Carrots
□□□□□□□	Corn
□□□□□□□	Parsnips
□□□□□□□	Peas (green)
□□□□□□□	Spinach
□□□□□□□	Sweet potatoes
□□□□□□□	Turnips

(2 to 4.4 g/serving, average 3.5 g/serving)

M T W T F S S	Fruits
□□□□□□□	Apricots, dried (10 halves)
□□□□□□□	Apples (1 fruit)
□□□□□□□	Avocado* (1 fruit)
□□□□□□□	Banana (1 fruit)
□□□□□□□	Blueberries
□□□□□□□	Cantaloupe (½ fruit)
□□□□□□□	Gooseberries
□□□□□□□	Mangoes (1 fruit)
□□□□□□□	Nectarines (1 fruit)
□□□□□□□	Oranges (1 fruit)
□□□□□□□	Pear, raw (1 fruit)
□□□□□□□	Raisins (40 ml)
□□□□□□□	Rhubarb, cooked
□□□□□□□	Raspberries
□□□□□□□	Strawberries

M T W T F S S	Nuts*
□□□□□□□	Almonds, unblanched (15 nuts)
□□□□□□□	Brazilnuts, unblanched, (5)
□□□□□□□	Walnuts (100 ml)
□□□□□□□	Filberts, unblanched (100 ml)
□□□□□□□	Peanut Butter (30 ml)

Thursday	Friday	Saturday	Sunday
□□□□	H □□□□	H □□□□	H □□□□
□□□□□□□□	M □□□□□□□□	M □□□□□□□□	M □□□□□□□□
__ servings × 5 = __ g	__ servings × 5 = __ g	__ servings × 5 = __ g	__ servings × 5 = __ g
__ servings × 3.5 = __ g	__ servings × 3.5 = __ g	__ servings × 3.5 = __ g	__ servings × 3.5 = __ g

TOTAL FIBRE PLANNER — *Week Nine*

High Sources

(4.5 g or more/serving, averaging 5 g/serving)

M T W T F S S   *Breads and Cereals*
☐☐☐☐☐☐☐ All Bran
☐☐☐☐☐☐☐ Bran Buds
☐☐☐☐☐☐☐ 100% Bran

M T W T F S S   *Legumes*
☐☐☐☐☐☐☐ Baked beans
☐☐☐☐☐☐☐ Kidney beans
☐☐☐☐☐☐☐ Dried peas and beans cooked

M T W T F S S   *Fruits*
☐☐☐☐☐☐☐ Dates (8)
☐☐☐☐☐☐☐ Dried figs (4)
☐☐☐☐☐☐☐ Prunes (5)

M T W T F S S   *Nuts**
☐☐☐☐☐☐☐ Peanuts (100 ml)

Moderate Sources

(2 to 4.4 g/serving, average 3.5 g/serving)

M T W T F S S   *Breads and Cereals*
☐☐☐☐☐☐☐ Bran Chex
☐☐☐☐☐☐☐ Bran Flakes
☐☐☐☐☐☐☐ Corn Bran
☐☐☐☐☐☐☐ Cracklin' Bran
☐☐☐☐☐☐☐ Fruit & Fibre
☐☐☐☐☐☐☐ Muffets
☐☐☐☐☐☐☐ Shredded Wheat
☐☐☐☐☐☐☐ Whole Wheat Bread (2 slices)
☐☐☐☐☐☐☐ Cracked Wheat Bread
(2 slices)
☐☐☐☐☐☐☐ Rye Bread (2 slices)
☐☐☐☐☐☐☐ Bran Muffins (1 small)
☐☐☐☐☐☐☐ Bulgar (cooked, 75 ml)

M T W T F S S   *Legumes*
☐☐☐☐☐☐☐ Lentils

Unless indicated all values are based upon 125 ml (½ cup) portions.

*High in fat. Don't use too often as a source of fibre.

DAILY RECORD

	Monday	Tuesday	Wednesday
High	☐☐☐☐	H ☐☐☐☐	H ☐☐☐☐
Moderate	☐☐☐☐☐☐☐	M ☐☐☐☐☐☐☐	M ☐☐☐☐☐☐☐
Totals (approx.)	_____	_____	_____
High	__ servings × 5 = __ g	__ servings × 5 = __ g	__ servings × 5 = __ g
Moderate	__ servings × 3.5 = __ g	__ servings × 3.5 = __ g	__ servings × 3.5 = __ g

(2 to 4.4 g/serving, average 3.5 g/serving)

M T W T F S S	Vegetables
□□□□□□□	Beets
□□□□□□□	Broccoli
□□□□□□□	Brussels Sprouts
□□□□□□□	Cabbage
□□□□□□□	Carrots
□□□□□□□	Corn
□□□□□□□	Parsnips
□□□□□□□	Peas (green)
□□□□□□□	Spinach
□□□□□□□	Sweet potatoes
□□□□□□□	Turnips

(2 to 4.4 g/serving, average 3.5 g/serving)

M T W T F S S	Fruits
□□□□□□□	Apricots, dried (10 halves)
□□□□□□□	Apples (1 fruit)
□□□□□□□	Avocado* (1 fruit)
□□□□□□□	Banana (1 fruit)
□□□□□□□	Blueberries
□□□□□□□	Cantaloupe (1/2 fruit)
□□□□□□□	Gooseberries
□□□□□□□	Mangoes (1 fruit)
□□□□□□□	Nectarines (1 fruit)
□□□□□□□	Oranges (1 fruit)
□□□□□□□	Pear, raw (1 fruit)
□□□□□□□	Raisins (40 ml)
□□□□□□□	Rhubarb, cooked
□□□□□□□	Raspberries
□□□□□□□	Strawberries

M T W T F S S	Nuts*
□□□□□□□	Almonds, unblanched (15 nuts)
□□□□□□□	Brazilnuts, unblanched, (5)
□□□□□□□	Walnuts (100 ml)
□□□□□□□	Filberts, unblanched (100 ml)
□□□□□□□	Peanut Butter (30 ml)

Thursday	Friday	Saturday	Sunday
H □□□□	H □□□□	H □□□□	H □□□□
M □□□□□□□	M □□□□□□□	M □□□□□□□	M □□□□□□□
__ servings × 5 = __ g	__ servings × 5 = __ g	__ servings × 5 = __ g	__ servings × 5 = __ g
__ servings × 3.5 = __ g	__ servings × 3.5 = __ g	__ servings × 3.5 = __ g	__ servings × 3.5 = __ g

TOTAL FIBRE PLANNER — *Week Ten*

High Sources

(4.5 g or more/serving, averaging 5 g/serving)

M T W T F S S	Breads and Cereals
☐☐☐☐☐☐☐	All Bran
☐☐☐☐☐☐☐	Bran Buds
☐☐☐☐☐☐☐	100% Bran

M T W T F S S	Legumes
☐☐☐☐☐☐☐	Baked beans
☐☐☐☐☐☐☐	Kidney beans
☐☐☐☐☐☐☐	Dried peas and beans cooked

M T W T F S S	Fruits
☐☐☐☐☐☐☐	Dates (8)
☐☐☐☐☐☐☐	Dried figs (4)
☐☐☐☐☐☐☐	Prunes (5)

M T W T F S S	Nuts*
☐☐☐☐☐☐☐	Peanuts (100 ml)

Moderate Sources

(2 to 4.4 g/serving, average 3.5 g/serving)

M T W T F S S	Breads and Cereals
☐☐☐☐☐☐☐	Bran Chex
☐☐☐☐☐☐☐	Bran Flakes
☐☐☐☐☐☐☐	Corn Bran
☐☐☐☐☐☐☐	Cracklin' Bran
☐☐☐☐☐☐☐	Fruit & Fibre
☐☐☐☐☐☐☐	Muffets
☐☐☐☐☐☐☐	Shredded Wheat
☐☐☐☐☐☐☐	Whole Wheat Bread (2 slices)
☐☐☐☐☐☐☐	Cracked Wheat Bread (2 slices)
☐☐☐☐☐☐☐	Rye Bread (2 slices)
☐☐☐☐☐☐☐	Bran Muffins (1 small)
☐☐☐☐☐☐☐	Bulgar (cooked, 75 ml)

M T W T F S S	Legumes
☐☐☐☐☐☐☐	Lentils

Unless indicated all values are based upon 125 ml (½ cup) portions.

*High in fat. Don't use too often as a source of fibre.

DAILY RECORD

	Monday	Tuesday	Wednesday
High	☐☐☐☐	H ☐☐☐☐	H ☐☐☐☐
Moderate	☐☐☐☐☐☐☐	M ☐☐☐☐☐☐☐	M ☐☐☐☐☐☐☐
Totals (approx.)	_____	_____	_____
High	__ servings × 5 = __ g	__ servings × 5 = __ g	__ servings × 5 = __ g
Moderate	__ servings × 3.5 = __ g	__ servings × 3.5 = __ g	__ servings × 3.5 = __ g

(2 to 4.4 g/serving, average 3.5 g/serving)

M T W T F S S	*Vegetables*
☐☐☐☐☐☐☐	Beets
☐☐☐☐☐☐☐	Broccoli
☐☐☐☐☐☐☐	Brussels Sprouts
☐☐☐☐☐☐☐	Cabbage
☐☐☐☐☐☐☐	Carrots
☐☐☐☐☐☐☐	Corn
☐☐☐☐☐☐☐	Parsnips
☐☐☐☐☐☐☐	Peas (green)
☐☐☐☐☐☐☐	Spinach
☐☐☐☐☐☐☐	Sweet potatoes
☐☐☐☐☐☐☐	Turnips

(2 to 4.4 g/serving, average 3.5 g/serving)

M T W T F S S	*Fruits*
☐☐☐☐☐☐☐	Apricots, dried (10 halves)
☐☐☐☐☐☐☐	Apples (1 fruit)
☐☐☐☐☐☐☐	Avocado* (1 fruit)
☐☐☐☐☐☐☐	Banana (1 fruit)
☐☐☐☐☐☐☐	Blueberries
☐☐☐☐☐☐☐	Cantaloupe (½ fruit)
☐☐☐☐☐☐☐	Gooseberries
☐☐☐☐☐☐☐	Mangoes (1 fruit)
☐☐☐☐☐☐☐	Nectarines (1 fruit)
☐☐☐☐☐☐☐	Oranges (1 fruit)
☐☐☐☐☐☐☐	Pear, raw (1 fruit)
☐☐☐☐☐☐☐	Raisins (40 ml)
☐☐☐☐☐☐☐	Rhubarb, cooked
☐☐☐☐☐☐☐	Raspberries
☐☐☐☐☐☐☐	Strawberries

M T W T F S S	*Nuts* *
☐☐☐☐☐☐☐	Almonds, unblanched (15 nuts)
☐☐☐☐☐☐☐	Brazilnuts, unblanched, (5)
☐☐☐☐☐☐☐	Walnuts (100 ml)
☐☐☐☐☐☐☐	Filberts, unblanched (100 ml)
☐☐☐☐☐☐☐	Peanut Butter (30 ml)

Thursday	Friday	Saturday	Sunday
H ☐☐☐☐	H ☐☐☐☐	H ☐☐☐☐	H ☐☐☐☐
M ☐☐☐☐☐☐☐	M ☐☐☐☐☐☐☐	M ☐☐☐☐☐☐☐	M ☐☐☐☐☐☐☐
___ servings × 5 = ___ g	___ servings × 5 = ___ g	___ servings × 5 = ___ g	___ servings × 5 = ___ g
___ servings × 3.5 = ___ g	___ servings × 3.5 = ___ g	___ servings × 3.5 = ___ g	___ servings × 3.5 = ___ g

TOTAL FIBRE PLANNER — *Week Eleven*

High Sources

(4.5 g or more/serving, averaging 5 g/serving)

M T W T F S S	Breads and Cereals
☐☐☐☐☐☐☐	All Bran
☐☐☐☐☐☐☐	Bran Buds
☐☐☐☐☐☐☐	100% Bran

M T W T F S S	Legumes
☐☐☐☐☐☐☐	Baked beans
☐☐☐☐☐☐☐	Kidney beans
☐☐☐☐☐☐☐	Dried peas and beans cooked

M T W T F S S	Fruits
☐☐☐☐☐☐☐	Dates (8)
☐☐☐☐☐☐☐	Dried figs (4)
☐☐☐☐☐☐☐	Prunes (5)

M T W T F S S	Nuts*
☐☐☐☐☐☐☐	Peanuts (100 ml)

Moderate Sources

(2 to 4.4 g/serving, average 3.5 g/serving)

M T W T F S S	Breads and Cereals
☐☐☐☐☐☐☐	Bran Chex
☐☐☐☐☐☐☐	Bran Flakes
☐☐☐☐☐☐☐	Corn Bran
☐☐☐☐☐☐☐	Cracklin' Bran
☐☐☐☐☐☐☐	Fruit & Fibre
☐☐☐☐☐☐☐	Muffets
☐☐☐☐☐☐☐	Shredded Wheat
☐☐☐☐☐☐☐	Whole Wheat Bread (2 slices)
☐☐☐☐☐☐☐	Cracked Wheat Bread (2 slices)
☐☐☐☐☐☐☐	Rye Bread (2 slices)
☐☐☐☐☐☐☐	Bran Muffins (1 small)
☐☐☐☐☐☐☐	Bulgar (cooked, 75 ml)

M T W T F S S	Legumes
☐☐☐☐☐☐☐	Lentils

Unless indicated all values are based upon 125 ml (½ cup) portions.

*High in fat. Don't use too often as a source of fibre.

DAILY RECORD

	Monday	Tuesday	Wednesday
High	☐☐☐☐	H ☐☐☐☐	H ☐☐☐☐
Moderate	☐☐☐☐☐☐	M ☐☐☐☐☐☐☐	M ☐☐☐☐☐☐☐
Totals (approx.)	_____	_____	_____
High	__ servings × 5 = __ g	__ servings × 5 = __ g	__ servings × 5 = __ g
Moderate	__ servings × 3.5 = __ g	__ servings × 3.5 = __ g	__ servings × 3.5 = __ g

(2 to 4.4 g/serving, average 3.5 g/serving)

M T W T F S S	Vegetables
☐☐☐☐☐☐☐	Beets
☐☐☐☐☐☐☐	Broccoli
☐☐☐☐☐☐☐	Brussels Sprouts
☐☐☐☐☐☐☐	Cabbage
☐☐☐☐☐☐☐	Carrots
☐☐☐☐☐☐☐	Corn
☐☐☐☐☐☐☐	Parsnips
☐☐☐☐☐☐☐	Peas (green)
☐☐☐☐☐☐☐	Spinach
☐☐☐☐☐☐☐	Sweet potatoes
☐☐☐☐☐☐☐	Turnips

(2 to 4.4 g/serving, average 3.5 g/serving)

M T W T F S S	Fruits
☐☐☐☐☐☐☐	Apricots, dried (10 halves)
☐☐☐☐☐☐☐	Apples (1 fruit)
☐☐☐☐☐☐☐	Avocado* (1 fruit)
☐☐☐☐☐☐☐	Banana (1 fruit)
☐☐☐☐☐☐☐	Blueberries
☐☐☐☐☐☐☐	Cantaloupe (½ fruit)
☐☐☐☐☐☐☐	Gooseberries
☐☐☐☐☐☐☐	Mangoes (1 fruit)
☐☐☐☐☐☐☐	Nectarines (1 fruit)
☐☐☐☐☐☐☐	Oranges (1 fruit)
☐☐☐☐☐☐☐	Pear, raw (1 fruit)
☐☐☐☐☐☐☐	Raisins (40 ml)
☐☐☐☐☐☐☐	Rhubarb, cooked
☐☐☐☐☐☐☐	Raspberries
☐☐☐☐☐☐☐	Strawberries

M T W T F S S	Nuts*
☐☐☐☐☐☐☐	Almonds, unblanched (15 nuts)
☐☐☐☐☐☐☐	Brazilnuts, unblanched, (5)
☐☐☐☐☐☐☐	Walnuts (100 ml)
☐☐☐☐☐☐☐	Filberts, unblanched (100 ml)
☐☐☐☐☐☐☐	Peanut Butter (30 ml)

Thursday	Friday	Saturday	Sunday
H ☐☐☐☐	H ☐☐☐☐	H ☐☐☐☐	H ☐☐☐☐
M ☐☐☐☐☐☐☐	M ☐☐☐☐☐☐☐	M ☐☐☐☐☐☐☐	M ☐☐☐☐☐☐☐

___ servings × 5 = ___ g   ___ servings × 5 = ___ g   ___ servings × 5 = ___ g   ___ servings × 5 = ___ g

___ servings × 3.5 = ___ g   ___ servings × 3.5 = ___ g   ___ servings × 3.5 = ___ g   ___ servings × 3.5 = ___ g

TOTAL FIBRE PLANNER — *Week Twelve*

High Sources

(4.5 g or more/serving, averaging 5 g/serving)

M T W T F S S	Breads and Cereals
☐☐☐☐☐☐☐	All Bran
☐☐☐☐☐☐☐	Bran Buds
☐☐☐☐☐☐☐	100% Bran

M T W T F S S	Legumes
☐☐☐☐☐☐☐	Baked beans
☐☐☐☐☐☐☐	Kidney beans
☐☐☐☐☐☐☐	Dried peas and beans cooked

M T W T F S S	Fruits
☐☐☐☐☐☐☐	Dates (8)
☐☐☐☐☐☐☐	Dried figs (4)
☐☐☐☐☐☐☐	Prunes (5)

M T W T F S S	Nuts*
☐☐☐☐☐☐☐	Peanuts (100 ml)

Moderate Sources

(2 to 4.4 g/serving, average 3.5 g/serving)

M T W T F S S	Breads and Cereals
☐☐☐☐☐☐☐	Bran Chex
☐☐☐☐☐☐☐	Bran Flakes
☐☐☐☐☐☐☐	Corn Bran
☐☐☐☐☐☐☐	Cracklin' Bran
☐☐☐☐☐☐☐	Fruit & Fibre
☐☐☐☐☐☐☐	Muffets
☐☐☐☐☐☐☐	Shredded Wheat
☐☐☐☐☐☐☐	Whole Wheat Bread (2 slices)
☐☐☐☐☐☐☐	Cracked Wheat Bread (2 slices)
☐☐☐☐☐☐☐	Rye Bread (2 slices)
☐☐☐☐☐☐☐	Bran Muffins (1 small)
☐☐☐☐☐☐☐	Bulgar (cooked, 75 ml)

M T W T F S S	Legumes
☐☐☐☐☐☐☐	Lentils

Unless indicated all values are based upon 125 ml (½ cup) portions.

*High in fat. Don't use too often as a source of fibre.

DAILY RECORD

	Monday	Tuesday	Wednesday
High	☐☐☐☐	H ☐☐☐☐	H ☐☐☐☐
Moderate	☐☐☐☐☐☐☐	M ☐☐☐☐☐☐☐	M ☐☐☐☐☐☐☐
Totals (approx.)	———————	———————	———————
High	__ servings × 5 = __ g	__ servings × 5 = __ g	__ servings × 5 = __ g
Moderate	__ servings × 3.5 = __ g	__ servings × 3.5 = __ g	__ servings × 3.5 = __ g

(2 to 4.4 g/serving, average 3.5 g/serving)

M T W T F S S	Vegetables
□□□□□□□	Beets
□□□□□□□	Broccoli
□□□□□□□	Brussels Sprouts
□□□□□□□	Cabbage
□□□□□□□	Carrots
□□□□□□□	Corn
□□□□□□□	Parsnips
□□□□□□□	Peas (green)
□□□□□□□	Spinach
□□□□□□□	Sweet potatoes
□□□□□□□	Turnips

(2 to 4.4 g/serving, average 3.5 g/serving)

M T W T F S S	Fruits
□□□□□□□	Apricots, dried (10 halves)
□□□□□□□	Apples (1 fruit)
□□□□□□□	Avocado* (1 fruit)
□□□□□□□	Banana (1 fruit)
□□□□□□□	Blueberries
□□□□□□□	Cantaloupe (½ fruit)
□□□□□□□	Gooseberries
□□□□□□□	Mangoes (1 fruit)
□□□□□□□	Nectarines (1 fruit)
□□□□□□□	Oranges (1 fruit)
□□□□□□□	Pear, raw (1 fruit)
□□□□□□□	Raisins (40 ml)
□□□□□□□	Rhubarb, cooked
□□□□□□□	Raspberries
□□□□□□□	Strawberries

M T W T F S S	Nuts*
□□□□□□□	Almonds, unblanched (15 nuts)
□□□□□□□	Brazilnuts, unblanched, (5)
□□□□□□□	Walnuts (100 ml)
□□□□□□□	Filberts, unblanched (100 ml)
□□□□□□□	Peanut Butter (30 ml)

Thursday	Friday	Saturday	Sunday
H □□□□	H □□□□	H □□□□	H □□□□
M □□□□□□□	M □□□□□□□	M □□□□□□□	M □□□□□□□
___ servings × 5 = ___ g	___ servings × 5 = ___ g	___ servings × 5 = ___ g	___ servings × 5 = ___ g
___ servings × 3.5 = ___ g	___ servings × 3.5 = ___ g	___ servings × 3.5 = ___ g	___ servings × 3.5 = ___ g

CHAPTER 10

HI-FI DIETING
Sounds easy, doesn't it?

*I*f the pendulum of life continues its back and forth motion, and if history indeed repeats itself, the time may exist once again when plumpness in ladies is admired as it was in the heyday of Reubens. "Pleasingly plump" might replace "glaringly gaunt" as a compliment, and models might even have a curve or two. But don't hold your breath.

And until society's notion of acceptable or desirable levels of adiposity is better reconciled with reality, the majority of the populace — both male and female — will most likely continue its love affair with the get-thin-quick fad diets and weight-loss gimmicks.

A recent entry into the girth-control sweepstakes highlights the problem. Called "the amino night diet," the wonder supplement is an assortment of amino acids (arginine and histidine are two biggies) and is reputed to alter one's hormones so that the body's metabolism resembles that of a teenager, and fat just melts away — all while you sleep! People tend to fall for this sales pitch, especially because amino acids are "natural." Not dished up like this, they're not!

Other substances that aren't quite so "natural," but nonetheless striving for popularity, are the timed-release "diet aids." Sold under various names but mostly containing a substance called phenylpropanolamine, these diet "pills" have actually been shown by some studies to be effective for SHORT TERM weight reduction. Interestingly enough, the amount of weight loss directly attributable to the drug itself has generally been quite small.

So how about the safety of the drug? Increase in blood pressure seems to be the major side effect, with severe hypertension and stroke possibly occurring with both recommended dosage and overdose. In addition to blood pressure problems, there have been reports of central nervous system disturbances, psychotic episodes, paranoia, homicidal behavior, hallucinations and attempted suicide after taking phenylpropanolamine. All this and weight loss too! PPA is also found on the "street" market, often in combination with other drugs as a substitute for amphetamine. Its abuse has been associated with acute renal failure and fatal cerebral hemorrhage. In summary, weight loss with these pills is usually small and maintained only as long as drug use is continued. There's no evidence of long-term effectiveness — and the side effects could be disastrous.

Does this mean that there's no help in the battle-of-the-bulge? Not exactly. While it's true that any sensible weight-loss plan involves a reduced intake of foods from Canada's Food Guide coupled with a sound exercise program, there is some evidence that fibre might make the battle less burdensome.

FIBRE AND WEIGHT LOSS
In the section on obesity in Chapter 5, we discussed the various ways that a high-fibre diet might lead to a lowered calorie intake by usurping the high-energy, fatty foods normally consumed. Not only would fibrous foods "push aside" low-nutrient, high-calorie foods, they would also provide a high

level of satiety while doing it. That's the theory, but are there any studies to support it?

One particularly interesting study of high-fibre diets for obese diabetic patients was conducted by J.A. Anderson and Beverly Sieling of the University of Kentucky College of Medicine. In their report in the journal *Obesity/Bariatric Medicine*, Volume 9, No. 4, 1980, Anderson and Sieling noted significantly lower insulin requirements, blood glucose and lipids in their patients following a calorie-restricted (600 to 1,000 calories), but high-fibre (32 to 50 grams of plant fibre) diet. They also noted significant weight loss with minimal hunger when the diet was high in fibre.

An excellent review on fibre and obesity by Theodore Van Itallie appeared in the October, 1978, issue of *The American Journal of Clinical Nutrition*. The workshop surmised that dietary fibre might prove an impediment to consumption of excessive calories in several ways, but emphasis was given to delayed gastric emptying, reduced caloric concentration of gastric contents (think of this as diluted), and increased volume of the substance in the small intestine, which could largely account for feelings of satiety.

At this point, the relevant factors relating to fibre and weight loss are still speculation, but there seems little doubt as to the end result: when a high-fibre diet is consumed, obesity is generally uncommon.

Given the acceptance of the above, one would naturally wonder: a) if people have used a high-fibre diet to help them lose weight, and b) whether a supplemental form of fibre such as Fibre Trim could be useful in shedding fat. Yes, one would — and all that wondering led to two interesting studies. The first appeared in *The Journal of the Norwegian Medical Association*, No. 24, 1983, and described the effects of dietary-fibre tablets in a group of 30 patients consuming an 1,100-calorie diet with approximately 30 grams of fibre. A control group (23) consumed the same diet but with the dietary-fibre tablets replaced by an equal number of placebo tablets. After eight weeks on the program, the fibre-tablet dieters had lost significantly more weight than their placebo-popping counterparts. But perhaps even more important, they didn't mind being on the diet and didn't feel hungry.

Please note two important points: both groups were consuming well-planned, nutritionally-balanced diets, and they were eating 1,100 calories per day. Anybody can lose weight by starving. It takes some discipline to adhere to a well-chosen meal plan.

The second study followed two groups of 45 women each in a weight-loss club, all of whom were at least 15 per cent over their ideal weight. This time, the diet consisted of 1,200 calories per day. Each day the women were given either seven fibre tablets like Fibre Trim (a mixture of cereal and citrus fruit fibres contributing 10 grams of dietary fibre) or seven placebo tablets. Two results are worthy of note: there was greater weight loss in the fibre-tablet group, and there was a significantly reduced tendency to discontinue the weight-loss program.

These studies in no way prove that fibre tablets cause one to burn off excess fat. What they seem to indicate is an increased ability to stay with a calorie-reduced program, thanks to a lessening of hunger. I've had several clients use fibre pills like Fibre Trim in conjunction with a nutritionally balanced diet plan, and all reported the same thing: "Stayed with it because I didn't feel hungry." There might be cause for concern with this type of product if someone decided to use the pills in order to eat as little as possible. There's a word for that: dumb.

There's no end of examples of people who have dieted inappropriately, subsisting on a minimum caloric intake, only to end up skinny, malnourished and unhealthy. To make matters worse, because their starvation regimen effectively lowered their basal metabolic rate (the minimum amount of energy you use just to keep on ticking), as soon as they started to eat halfway normally (pigging out on maybe 1,200 calories), they regained all their lost weight plus a little extra. And why? Because metabolic rate was decreased. Hence the yo-yo effect.

If you want to lose weight, make up your mind that this time you're going to be smart about it. Try the program here — high in fibre and nutrients and low in fat, but providing roughly 1,200 calories so your body won't go into a state-of-siege attitude. If you have trouble with hunger pains, you might find fibre pills like Fibre Trim to be of help. They won't hurt and they won't promise you instant or eternal slimhood. Fat loss is never easy. This plan may just be a little less burdensome than most.

SEVEN DAY WEIGHT-REDUCTION PLAN

High in fibre, low in fat — 1200 to 1250 calories

Breakfast	Lunch	Dinner

Day 1

1 large shredded wheat biscuit
1 cup (250 mL) skim milk
1 banana
	pita stuffed with
	   ½ cup (125 mL) shredded
	   cabbage
	   1 raw carrot shredded
	   2 oz chicken
	   1 tbsp (15 mL) vinaigrette
	   dressing (see page 120)
	1 orange
	1 cup (250 mL) skim milk
		3 oz (90 g) well trimmed lean roast
		   beef
		Baked Potato Primavera
		   (see page 127)
		broccoli with lemon juice
		1 pear

Calories 1232   **Dietary Fibre** 23.7 gm   **Calories from fat** 16.3%

Day 2

½ cantaloupe
1 Blueberry Bran Muffin without
   topping (see page 145)
1 oz (30 gm) part skim mozzarella
   cheese
	2 slices rye bread
	1 slice very lean ham
	⅓ cup (80 mL) sauerkraut
	2 tsp (10 mL) mustard
	½ cup (125 mL) grapes
	1 cup (250 mL) skim milk
		Jellied Gazpacho (see page 101)
		2 eggs scrambled in a no-stick pan
		   with ¼ cup (60 mL) alfalfa
		   sprouts and 1 tbsp (15 mL)
		   sunflower seeds
		Banana Coconut Bread
		   (see page 151)
		1 cup (250 mL) skim milk

Calories 1217   **Dietary Fibre** 13.96 gm   **Calories from fat** 28.7%

Day 3

½ grapefruit
1 cup (250 mL) raisin bran
1 cup (250 mL) skim milk
	½ cup (125 mL) 2% cottage cheese
	½ cup (125 mL) fruit salad
	1 slice whole wheat bread
	1 tsp (5 mL) margarine
		Baked Beans (see page 118)
		No-Knead Oatmeal Batter Bread
		   (see page 146)
		Greens and Fruit with Curry
		   Vinaigrette (see page 98)
		½ cup (125 mL) plain 2% yogurt

Calories 1225   **Dietary Fibre** 23.35 gm   **Calories from fat** 26.2%

Day 4

½ cup (125 mL) orange juice
1 slice whole wheat toast
½ cup (125 mL) 2% cottage cheese
6 dried apricot halves

Pumpernickel Caraway Bread (see page 140)
2 oz (60 gm) sliced chicken
spinach salad
   with 1 tbsp (15 mL) low-cal Italian dressing
1 cup (250 mL) skim milk

Company Chili (see page 119)
2 Caraway Crisps (see page 143)
Refrigerator Coleslaw (see page 105)
½ cup (125 mL) unsweetened blueberries
1 cup (250 mL) skim milk

Calories   1234   **Dietary Fibre**   26.3 gm   **Calories from fat**   22.1%

Day 5

¾ cup (175 mL) oatmeal
1 peach half
1 cup (250 mL) skim milk

Split Pea Soup (see page 95)
1 Whole Wheat Biscuit (see page 141)
1 tsp (5 mL) butter
1 apple
1 cup (250 mL) skim milk

Saucy Ginger-Baked Fish (see page 123)
1 medium boiled potato
1 tsp (5 mL) butter
½ cup (125 mL) turnip
Raspberry Yogurt Mould (see page 164)

Calories   1212   **Dietary Fibre**   27.4 gm   **Calories from fat**   22.4%

Day 6

½ cup (125 mL) grapefruit juice
½ cup (125 mL) plain 2% yogurt
1 small bran muffin
5 cooked prunes (no added sugar)

Pasta Niçoise (see page 103)
1 apple
1 cup (250 mL) skim milk

3 oz (90 gm) very lean pork
½ cup (125 mL) brown rice
2 tbsp (30 mL) applesauce
Lima Bean Bake (see page 115)
½ cup (125 mL) unsweetened raspberries
½ cup (125 mL) skim milk

Calories   1247   **Dietary Fibre**   21.0 gm   **Calories from fat**   20.6%

Day 7

1 orange
2 Double Corn Pancakes (see page 126)
low-cal syrup

Mix-and-Match Vegetable Soup (see page 94)
Stir-Fried Spinach with Lentils (see page 131)
Zucchini Wheat Germ Bread (see page 152)
1 cup (250 mL) skim milk

Mushroom Barley Bake (see page 133)
1 small baked sweet potato
½ cup (125 mL) brussel sprouts
½ cup (125 mL) unsweetened strawberries
1 cup (250 mL) skim milk

Calories   1230   **Dietary Fibre**   27.7 gm   **Calories from fat**   22.2%

Summary

The calories for this seven-day meal plan range from 1212 to 1247. Except for the 2nd day the dietary fibre is over 20 gm per day. The calories from fat are always under 30 per cent.

This seven-day meal plan meets the "Recommended Nutrient Intake for Canadian Women 19 to 49 Years" for all nutrients with the exception of iron (average daily value = 11.6 gm vs a requirement of 14 gm). Zinc may also be low; however, the amount present is consistent with the finding that the mixed Canadian diet provides about 5 mg of zinc per 1000 kcal. ("Recommended Nutrient Intakes for Canadians", Health and Welfare Canada, 1983.)

YOUR FINAL QUIZ ON FIBRE

MULTIPLE CHOICE

1. A common dietary problem with children is
   a) anything that's green makes them sick
   b) their typically "favorite" foods are low in fibre
   c) their moms won't make macaroni dinner for breakfast
   d) they eat too much liver, which has no fibre

2. A common dietary problem for the elderly is
   a) the kids get all the good stuff
   b) teeth stored in a glass can't handle corn-on-the-cob
   c) inadequate fluid intake
   d) too many prune jokes

3. Besides providing fibre, carrots
   a) enabled Superman to see through buildings
   b) ensured Bugs Bunny's dominance over Elmer Fudd
   c) provide significant amounts of retinol
   d) provide significant amounts of carotene

4. Polished rice is a good source of
   a) not much
   b) vitamin B_6
   c) beri-beri
   d) cyanocobalamin

5. Baked beans are an excellent source of
   a) fibre
   b) protein
   c) embarrassment
   d) all of the above

6. An incomplete protein
   a) hasn't found a mate
   b) is lacking one or more of the essential amino acids
   c) has no purpose in life
   d) contains insufficient iron

7. Guar gum is a type of
   a) seaweed
   b) fibre
   c) glue
   d) rock group

8. Diverticulosis is a form of
   a) outpouchings on the bowel wall
   b) bad breath
   c) appendicitis
   d) gastric upset

9. Beta glucans is a cholesterol-lowering substance found in
   a) French fries
   b) spinach
   c) Big Macs
   d) oat bran

10. People who are over-fat should
    a) enjoy themselves anyway
    b) replace fatty foods with high-fibre foods
    c) concentrate on their inner beauty
    d) follow the grapefruit diet

Answers: 1(b); 2(c); 3(d); 4(a); 5(d); 6(b); 7(b); 8(a); 9(d); 10(b) with (a) and (c) runners-up. (This was a trick question.)

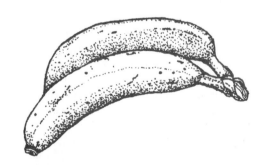

BIBLIOGRAPHY

Anderson, B.M., Gibson, R.S. and Sabry, J.H. "The Iron and Zinc Status of Long-term Vegetarian Women." *American Journal of Clinical Nutrition* 34:1042-1048, 1981.

Anderson, J.W. and Chen, W.-J.L. "Plant Fiber. Carbohydrate and Lipid Metabolism." *American Journal of Clinical Nutrition* 32:346-363, 1979.

Anderson, J.W. and Sieling, B. "High-fibre Diets for Obese Diabetic Patients." *Obesity/ Bariatric Medicine* 9:109-113, 1980.

Anderson, J.W. and Ward, K. "High-carbohydrate, High-fibre Diets for Insulin-treated Men with Diabetes Mellitus." *American Journal of Clinical Nutrition* 32:2312-2321, 1979.

Anderson, J.W., Ferguson, S.K., Karounos, D., O'Malley, L., Sieling, B., Chen, W.-J.L. "Mineral and Vitamin Status on High-fibre Diets: Long-term Studies of Diabetic Patients." *Diabetes Care* 3,1:38-40, 1980.

Anderson, J.W., Story, L., Sieling, B., Chen, W.-J.L., Petro, M.S., Story, J. "Hypocholesterolemic Effects of Oat-bran or Bean Intake for Hypercholesterolemic Men." *American Journal of Clinical Nutrition*, 40,6:1146-1155, 1984.

Blackburn, N.A., Redfern, J.S., Jarjis, H., Holgate, A.M., Hanning, I., Scarpello, J.H.B., Johnson, I.T., Read, N.W. "The Mechanism of Action of Guar Gum in Improving Glucose Tolerance in Man." *Clinical Science* 66:329-336, 1984.

Bolton, R.P., Heaton, K.W., Burroughs, L.F. "The Role of Dietary Fibre in Satiety, Glucose and Insulin: Studies with Fruit and Fruit Juices." *American Journal of Clinical Nutrition* 34:211-217, 1981.

Burkitt, D.P., Walker, A.R.P., Painter, N.S. "Dietary Fiber and Disease." *Journal of the American Medical Association* 229:1068-1074, 1974.

Cummings, J.H. "Short Chain Fatty Acids in the Human Colon." *Gut* 22:763-779, 1981.

Cummings, J.H. "Fermentation in the Human Large Intestine: Evidence and Implications for Health." *Lancet* 1:1206-1208, 1983.

Cummings, J.H., Hill, M.J., Jenkins, D.J.A., Pearson, J.R., Wiggins, H.S. "Changes in Fecal Composition and Colonic Function due to Cereal Fiber." *American Journal of Clinical Nutrition* 29:1468-1473, 1976.

Cummings, J.H., Branch, W.J., Bjerrum, L., Paerregaard, A., Helms, P., Burton, R. "Colon Cancer and Large Bowel Function in Denmark and Finland." *Nutrition and Cancer* 4,1:61-66, 1982.

Eastwood, M.A. and Kay, R.M. "An Hypothesis for the Action of Dietary Fiber along the Gastrointestinal Tract." *American Journal of Clinical Nutrition* 32:364-367, 1979.

Eastwood, M.A., Kirkpatrick, J.R., Mitchell, W.D., Bone, A., Hamilton, T. "Effects of Dietary Supplements of Wheat Bran and Cellulose and Faeces and Bowel Function." *British Medical Journal* 4:392-394, 1973.

Ehle, F.R., Robertson, J.B., Van Soest, P.J. "Influence of Dietary Fibers on Fermentation in the Human Large Intestine." *Journal of Nutrition* 112:158-166, 1982.

Gibson, R.S. and Scythes, C.A. "Trace Element Intakes of Women." *British Journal of Nutrition* 48:241-248, 1981.

Graham, D.Y., Moser, S.E., Estes, M.K. "The Effect of Bran on Bowel Function in Constipation." *American Journal of Gastroenterology* 77,9:599-603, 1982.

Grahams, S., Dayal, H., Swanson, M., et al. "Diet in the Epidemiology of Cancer of the Colon and Rectum." *Journal of the National Cancer Institute* 61:709-714, 1978.

Haber, G.B., Heaton, K.W., Murphy, D., Burroughs, L.F. "Depletion and Disruption of Dietary Fibre: Effects on Satiety, Plasma Glucose and Serum Insulin." *Lancet* 2:679, 1977.

Heaton, K.W. "Food Fibre as an Obstacle to Energy Intake." *Lancet* 2:1418, 1973.

Heaton, K.W. "Is Bran Useful in Diverticular Disease?" *British Medical Journal* 283:1523-1524, 1981.

Hylander, B. and Rossner, S. "Effects of Dietary Fiber Intake Before Meals on Weight Loss and Hunger in a Weight-reducing Club." *Acta Med Scand* 213:217-220, 1983.

Jenkins, D.J.A. "Lente Carbohydrate: A Newer Approach to the Dietary Management of Diabetes." *Diabetes Care* 5,6:634-641, 1982.

Jenkins, D.J.A., Leeds, A.R., Gassull, M.A., Wolever, T.M.S., Goff, D.V., Alberti, K.G.M.M. "Unabsorbable Carbohydrates and Diabetes: Decreased Postprandial Hyperglycemia." *Lancet* 2:172-174, 1976.

Jenkins, D.J.A., Leeds, A.R., Gassull, M.A., Cochet, B., Alberti K.G.M.M. "Decrease in Postprandial Insulin and Glucose Concentrations by Guar and Pectin." *Annals of Internal Medicine* 86:20-23, 1977a.

Jenkins, D.J.A., Wolever, T.M.S., Leeds, A.R., Gassull, M.A., Haisman, P., Dilawari, J., Goff, D.V., Metz, G.L., Alberti, K.G.M.M. "Dietary Fibers, Fiber Analogues, and Glucose Tolerance: Importance of Viscosity." *British Medical Journal* 1:1392-1394, 1978a.

Jenkins, D.J.A., Leeds, A.R., Slavin, B., Mann, J., Jenson, E.M. "Dietary Fiber and Blood Lipids: Reduction of Serum Cholesterol in Type II Hyperlipidemia by Guar Gum." *American Journal of Clinical Nutrition* 32:16-18, 1979a.

Jenkins, D.J.A., Wolever, T.M.S., Taylor, R.H., Barker, H.M., Fielden, H., Jenkins, A.L. "Effect of Guar Crispbread with Cereal Products and Leguminous Seeds on Blood Glucose Concentrations of Diabetics." *British Medical Journal* 281:1248-50, 1980b.

Jenkins, D.J.A., Wolever, T.M.S., Taylor, R.H., Barker, H., Fielden, H., Baldwin, J.M., Bowling, A.C., Newman, H.C., Jenkins, A.L., Goff, D.V. "Glycemic Index of Foods: A Physiological Basis for Carbohydrate Exchange." *American Journal of Clinical Nutrition* 34:362-366, 1981.

Jenkins, D.J.A., Wong, G.S., Patten, R., Bird, J., Hall, M., Buckley, G.C., McGuire, V., Reichert, R., Little, J.A. "Leguminous Seeds in the Dietary Management of Hyperlipidemia." *American Journal of Clinical Nutrition* 38:567-573, 1983b.

Kay, R.M. "Dietary Fiber." *Journal of Lipid Research* 23:221-242, 1982.

Kay, R.M. and Truswell, A.S. "Effect of Citrus Pectin on Blood Lipids and Fecal Steroid Excretion in Man." *American Journal of Clinical*

Nutrition 30:171-175, 1977.

Kelsay, J.L. "Effect of Dietary Fibre Level on Bowel Function and Trace Mineral Balances of Human Subjects." *Cereal Chemistry* 58,1:2-5, 1981.

Kelsay, J.L., Clark, W.M., Herbst, B.J., Prather, E.S. "Nutrient Utilization by Human Subjects Consuming Fruits and Vegetables as Sources of Fiber." *Journal of Agricultural Food Chemistry* 29:461-465, 1981.

Keys, A., Grande, F., Anderson, J.T. "Fiber and Pectin in the Diet and Serum Cholesterol Concentration in Man." *Proceedings of the Society of Experimental Biological Medicine* 106:555-558, 1961.

Kritchevsky, D. "Fiber, Lipids, and Atherosclerosis." *American Journal of Clinical Nutrition* 31:565-574, 1978.

Kritchevsky, D. and Story, J.A. "Binding of Bile Salts in Vitro by Nonnutritive Fiber." *Journal of Nutrition* 104:458-462, 1974.

Miettinen, T.A. and Tarpila, S. "Effect of Pectin on Serum Cholesterol, Fecal Bile Acids and Biliary Lipids in Normolipidemic and Hyperlipidemic Individuals." *Clin Chim Acta* 79:471-477, 1977.

McCance, R.D., Widdowson, O. "Old Thought and New Work on Breads White and Brown." *Lancet* 2:205-210, 1955.

Ohi, G., Minowa, K., Oyoma, T., et al. "Changes in Dietary Fiber Intake among Japanese in the 20th Century: A Relationship to the Prevalence of Diverticular Disease." *American Journal of Clinical Nutrition* 38,1:115-121, 1983.

Painter, N.S. and Burkitt, D.P. "Diverticular Disease of the Colon: A Deficiency Disease of Western Civilization." *British Medical Journal* 2:450-454, 1971.

Painter, N.S., Almeida, A.Z., Colebourne, K.W. "Unprocessed Bran in Treatment of Diverticular Disease of the Colon." *British Medical Journal* 2:137-140, 1972.

Payler, D.K., Pomare, E.W., Heaton, K.W., Harvey, R.F. "The Effect of Wheat Bran on Intestinal Transit." *Gut* 16:209-213, 1975.

Prosky, L., Asp, N.G., Furda, I., DeVries, J.W., Schweizer, T.F., Harland, B.F. "Determination of Total Dietary Fiber in Foods and Food Products: Collaborative Study."

Journal of the Association of Analytical Chemistry 68,4:677-679, 1985.

Reinhold, J.G., Lahimgarzadeh, A., Nasr, K., Hedayati, H. "Effects of Purified Phytate and Phytate-rich Bread upon Metabolism of Zinc, Calcium, Phosphorus and Nitrogen in Man." *Lancet* 1:283-288m, 1973.

Reinhold, J.G., Faradji, B., Abadi, P., Ismail-Beigi, F. "Decreased Absorption of Calcium, Magnesium, Zinc and Phosphorus by Humans due to Increased Fiber and Phosphorus Consumption as Wheat Bran." *Journal of Nutrition* 106:493-503, 1976.

Shah, B.G. "Bioavailability of Trace Elements in Human Nutrition." *Nutrition in Health and Disease and International Development: Symposia from the XII International Congress of Nutrition,* 1981. Alan R. Liss Inc., New York, pp. 199-208.

Simpson, H.C.R., Simpson, R.W., Lousley, S., Carter, R.D., Geekie, M., Hockaday, T.D.R., Mann, J.I. "A High-carbohydrate Leguminous Fibre Diet Improves All Aspects of Diabetic Control." *Lancet* 1:1-5, 1981a.

Southgate, D.A.T. "Determination of Carbohydrates in Foods II. Unavailable Carbohydrates." *Journal of Scientific Food and Agriculture* 20:331-335, 1969.

Southgate, D.A.T., Hudson, G.J., Englyst, H.

"The Analysis of Dietary Fibre: The Choices for the Analyst." *Journal of Scientific Food and Agriculture* 29:979-988, 1978.

Trowell, H., Southgate, D.A.T., Wolever, T.M.S., Leeds, A.R., Gassull, M.A., Jenkins, D.J.A. "Dietary Fibre Redefined." *Lancet* 1:967, 1976.

Valle-Jones, J.C. "The Evaluation of a New Appetite-Reducing Agent (Prefil) in the Management of Obesity." *British Journal of Clinical Practice* 34,3:72-74, 1980.

Van Itallie, T.B. "Dietary Fiber and Obesity." *American Journal of Clinical Nutrition* 31:S43-S52, 1978.

Van Soest, P.J. "Some Physical Characteristics of Dietary Fibres and Their Influence on the Microbial Ecology of the Human Colon." *Proceedings of the Nutrition Society* 43:25-33, 1984.

Van Soest, P.J. and Robertson, J.B. "What is Fibre and Fibre in Food?" *Nutrition Review* 35:12-22, 1977.

Wrick, K.L., Robertson, J.B., Van Soest, P.J., Lewis, B.A., Rivers, J.M., Roe, D.A., Hackler, L.R. "The Influence of Dietary Fiber Source on Human Intestinal Transit and Stool Output." *Journal of Nutrition* 113:1464-1479, 1983.

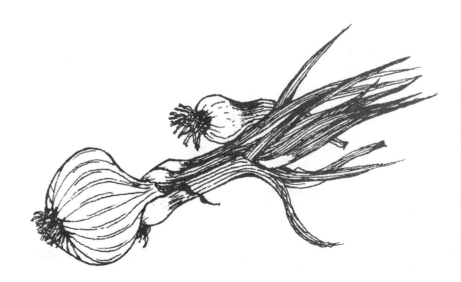

Fabulous Fibre Recipes

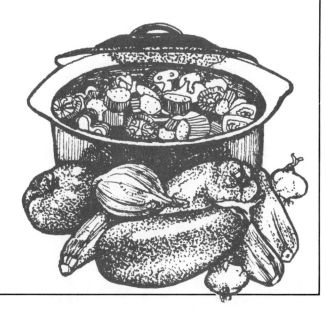

Acknowledgements

My thanks to Grosvenor House Press and to

— Bonnie Cowan and Arlene Lappin of *Canadian Living*
  magazine for encouraging me to do the recipes for this
  book.
— Karen Hanley, who kept us on track as a super editorial
  project coordinator.
— Carol Ferguson and Judy Brandow of *Canadian Living*
  magazine for allowing me to adapt some of my recipes
  previously published in the magazine.
— Sharyn Joliat of Info Access for scurrying to put my
  recipes through the computer for nutritional analysis.
— Ann Lindsay, author of *Smart Cooking*, for advice and
  encouragement.
— Fred Bird, food photographer extraordinaire, and
  Jennifer McLagan, a wonderful food stylist, for giving
  the food photographs a special touch of creativity.
— Bev Renahan for her great editing and careful typing,
  but most of all for her patience and encouragement.
— and to my husband Gil for tolerating both me and a lot of
  fibre through a short, hectic period of time!

Margaret Fraser
January 1987.

*I*NTRODUCTION

Creating the recipes on the following pages was a challenge but fun. There are scores of recipes high in fibre, but because it was not possible to include *all* the wonderful ones, it seemed more important to give a wide cross-section to show you the kinds of foods that contain lots of fibre, and are easy to prepare.

While trying to put as much fibre into each serving as possible, the goal was always a finished dish with both good taste and eye-appeal. The guidelines set out by the Canadian Cancer Society have been followed as closely as possible, although several good sources of fibre (like nuts) are also high in fat. When including foods of this nature in your meal-planning, try to reduce fat in other foods eaten during the day.

Suggestions have been made with some recipes to help you plan healthy meals. Preparation times are merely guidelines. One wheat sheaf indicates a moderate source of fibre (2 to 4.5 g), and two or three indicate a high source (4.6 to 6.9 g and 7 g or more). Follow Canada's Food Guide to ensure wise eating (see page 174).

Each recipe gives you the number of calories, grams of fat and fibre and a rating of vitamins and minerals per serving. Remember in your planning for good health you need, each day...

— 25 to 40 grams fibre
— adequate protein, about 15% of total calories
— fat not to exceed 30% of total calories
— 8 to 10 glasses of water or other liquids, such as juices, soup, beverages

All recipes were tested and analyzed using 2% milk, 2% yogurt, 2% cottage cheese, butter (because I prefer its flavor—but margarine may be used in its place) and 7% light sour cream. To ensure easy removal (and quick clean-ups), and to avoid any extra fat, I use a nonstick skillet and a generous spraying of low-calorie pure vegetable coating (like Pam) on baking surfaces.

Appetizers and Snacks

Grouped together, these two kinds of foods are much the same: small bites to tide you over, to nibble on before or between meals.

While usually full of flavor, whether savory or sweet, these tidbits served as munchies are often either loaded with fat (real calorie killers) or foods that have nothing but empty calories, that is, nutritionally poor. We've tried to make our appetizers and snacks as nutritionally perfect as possible. Each has added fibre to leave you feeling guilt-free after snacking. Where possible, forget the chips and serve fresh fruits or vegetables as dippers. Crackers should be made with whole-grain flours.

Remember, whether planning finger foods for parties or afternoon tea, kids' after-school treats or evening snacks, make them delicious as well as eye-appealing. Serve only enough to take the edge off appetites without over-indulging.

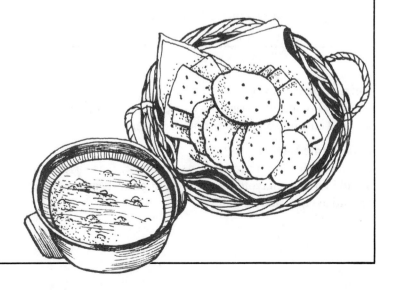

MEXICAN PARTY DIP

Preparation time: 20 minutes

*F*or a stunning platter, layer this spread in a 10- or 9-inch (25 or 23 cm) quiche dish. Centre it on a large tray and surround the dip with tortilla chips or crudités such as carrot slices, white turnip sticks or jicama, a Mexican vegetable now available in Canada.

Refried Bean Layer:

1	can (14 oz/398 mL) refried beans	1
1/4 cup	plain yogurt	50 mL
1/2 tsp	hot pepper flakes	2 mL
1/4 tsp	salt	1 mL
1/4 tsp	ground cumin	1 mL

Guacamole Layer:

1	ripe avocado, peeled and chopped	1
1/4 cup	finely chopped onion	50 mL
2 tbsp	mayonnaise	25 mL
1 tbsp	lemon juice	15 mL
Pinch	cayenne pepper	Pinch

Garnish:

1/3 cup	plain yogurt	75 mL
1/3 cup	sour cream	75 mL
2 cups	shredded Cheddar or Monterey Jack cheese	500 mL
5	green onions, sliced	5
1/2 cup	sliced pitted black olives	125 mL
2	tomatoes, chopped	2

Refried Bean Layer:
☐ Blend together refried beans, yogurt, hot pepper flakes, salt and cumin; spread over bottom of serving dish or tray.

Guacamole Layer:
☐ In blender, food processor or with fork, mash avocado; blend in onion, mayonnaise, lemon juice and cayenne. Spread over refried bean layer.

Garnish:

☐ Blend yogurt with sour cream; smooth lightly over guacamole layer. Sprinkle cheese in a ring around edge of dish. Make a ring of green onion slices inside cheese ring, then a ring of black olive slices. Place chopped tomatoes in centre. Refrigerate until serving time.

Makes 8 servings.

Calories per serving: 267   Excellent source of: Vitamin A
Grams fat per serving: 17.5   Good source of: Vitamin C,
Grams fibre per serving: 2.3   phosphorus and calcium

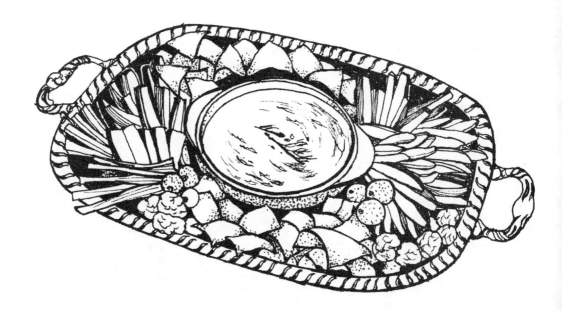

BROCCOLI DIP

Preparation time: 15 minutes

A perky basket of crudités surrounding this dip makes an attractive presentation. Serve cauliflower florets, red and green pepper strips, fresh yellow and green beans, and waffle-cut carrot slices.

2 cups	chopped broccoli	500 mL
2 tbsp	butter	25 mL
1	clove garlic, minced	1
2 cups	chopped mushrooms	500 mL
1/4 cup	chopped onion	50 mL
4 oz	light cream cheese	125 g
1/2 cup	Mock Sour Cream	125 mL
	Salt and freshly ground pepper	

To make **Mock Sour Cream:** In blender or food processor, combine 1 cup (250 mL) 2% cottage cheese, 1 tbsp (15 mL) each lemon juice and milk. Process until smooth. Store in refrigerator. Makes 1 cup (250 mL).

☐ Cook broccoli for 5 to 6 minutes or just until barely tender; drain and set aside.

☐ In skillet, melt butter over medium-high heat; cook garlic, mushrooms and onion for about 5 minutes or until onion is softened. Remove from heat.

☐ In food processor (or by hand), cream together cheese and Mock Sour Cream. Add broccoli and mushroom mixture; process until smooth. Season with salt and pepper to taste. Refrigerate until serving time.

Makes 2 cups (500 mL), or 6 servings.

Calories per serving: 103
Grams fat per serving: 7.5
Grams fibre per serving: 2

Excellent source of: Vitamin C
Good source of: Vitamin A

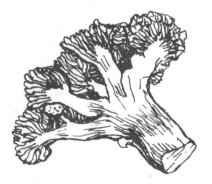

CHICK-PEA SPREAD

Preparation time: 10 minutes

*W*hole wheat crackers, melba toast or bread sticks are good accompaniments for this spread. Thick, diagonally sliced carrots, white turnip rounds or zucchini slices also go well and add a nice crunch.

1	can (19 oz/540 mL) chick-peas, drained and rinsed	1
2 tbsp	finely chopped green onion	25 mL
1	clove garlic, minced	1
2 tbsp	lemon juice	25 mL
2 tbsp	vegetable oil	25 mL
2 tbsp	chili sauce	25 mL
1 tsp	Dijon mustard	5 mL
1/4 tsp	salt	1 mL
2 tbsp	chopped fresh parsley	25 mL

Chick-Pea Spread is delicious spooned into croustades and topped with sliced stuffed olives. To make croustades: Cut 3-inch (8 cm) squares from thin slices of white or whole wheat bread. Flatten each square lightly with rolling pin and fit into 2-inch (5 cm) tart pans. Brush lightly with vegetable oil or melted butter. Bake in 350°F (180°C) oven for about 10 minutes or until lightly toasted. Remove from pans and let cool.

☐ In food processor, combine chick-peas, onion, garlic, lemon juice, oil, chili sauce, mustard and salt; process until smooth. Transfer to serving dish. Garnish with parsley. Chill until serving time.

Makes 2 cups (500 mL), or 8 servings.

Calories per serving: 102
Grams fat per serving: 4.2
Grams fibre per serving: 2.9

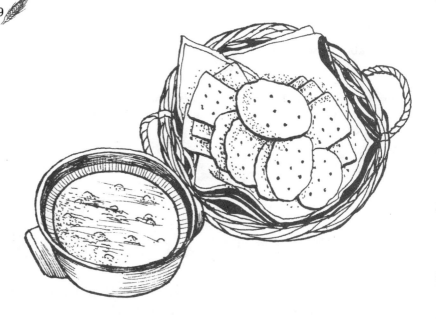

MARINATED BRUSSELS SPROUTS

Preparation time: 15 minutes
Chilling time: 3 hours

*O*ffer these with drinks before dinner, as part of an antipasto assortment or as an alternative to pickles. Store them in the refrigerator for up to one week.

1 lb	**Brussels sprouts**	500 g
2/3 cup	**vegetable oil**	150 mL
1/4 cup	**chopped fresh parsley**	50 mL
1/4 cup	**sliced green onions**	50 mL
1/4 cup	**tarragon or cider vinegar**	50 mL
1	**clove garlic, minced**	1
1 tsp	**ground marjoram**	5 mL
1/2 tsp	**salt**	2 mL
1/4 tsp	**coarse cracked black pepper**	1 mL

☐ In saucepan of boiling water, cook Brussels sprouts just until tender-crisp, about 10 minutes.

☐ Meanwhile, in blender or food processor, combine oil, parsley, green onions, vinegar, garlic, marjoram, salt and pepper; process until vegetables are finely chopped.

☐ Drain Brussels sprouts and refresh under cold running water to stop cooking; drain again and place in container. Pour marinade over; cover and marinate in refrigerator for several hours or overnight. To serve, remove sprouts with slotted spoon.

Makes about 6 servings.

Calories per serving: 74
Grams fat per serving: 5.1
Grams fibre per serving: 2.5

Excellent source of: Vitamin C
Good source of: Vitamin A

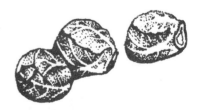

CHICKEN SATAY WITH PEANUT SAUCE

Preparation time: 10 minutes
Marinating time: 4 hours or
overnight
Cooking time: 8 minutes

*F*lavors of Southeast Asia make this sweet but hot appetizer appealing. Serve these with a red or white sangria or fruit punch.

4	boneless skinless chicken breasts (about 1-1/4 lb/625 g)	4
1/4 cup	finely chopped almonds	50 mL
1/4 cup	packed brown sugar	50 mL
2 tsp	soy sauce	10 mL
2	cloves garlic, crushed	2
2 tsp	coriander seeds, crushed	10 mL
1 tsp	fennel seeds	5 mL
1/8 tsp	crushed hot pepper flakes	0.5 mL
2 tbsp	sherry or chicken stock	25 mL
Sauce:		
1/2 cup	dry-roasted unsalted peanuts, finely chopped	125 mL
1/2 cup	peanut butter	125 mL
1/3 cup	water or chicken stock	75 mL
1 tsp	chili paste	5 mL

When barbecuing or broiling anything on bamboo or wooden skewers, soak the skewers in water for at least 30 minutes to prevent scorching or burning of the skewers.

☐ Cut chicken into 3/4-inch (2 cm) wide strips. In bowl, mix together almonds, brown sugar, soy sauce, garlic, coriander and fennel seeds and hot pepper flakes. Add chicken and sherry; mix well. Marinate chicken in refrigerator for at least 4 hours or overnight, stirring occasionally.

☐ Thread chicken onto soaked bamboo skewers, reserving marinade. Broil or barbecue skewers for about 4 minutes on each side or until chicken is tender but not dry, turning skewers once and basting occasionally with reserved marinade.

Sauce:

☐ Meanwhile, in small saucepan, mix together peanuts, peanut butter, water and chili paste; bring to simmer, adding some of the reserved marinade if sauce is too thick. Simmer for 3 minutes to blend flavors. Spoon over chicken or roll skewers in sauce.

Makes 8 appetizer servings.

Calories per serving: 278   Excellent source of: Niacin
Grams fat per serving: 16.3   Good source of: Phosphorus
Grams fibre per serving: 2.5

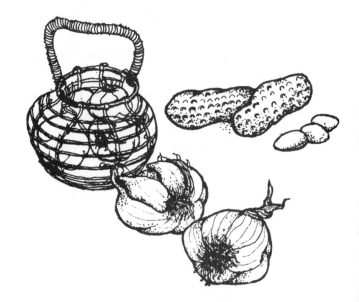

SNACKING SQUARES

Preparation time: 15 minutes
Baking time: 35 minutes

For a change of pace, use shredded unpeeled zucchini in place of carrots. Use 1/4 cup (50 mL) toasted sesame seeds instead of nuts or sunflower seeds.

1/2 cup	butter	125 mL
1 cup	lightly packed brown sugar	250 mL
1 tsp	vanilla	5 mL
1/4 tsp	freshly grated nutmeg	1 mL
2	eggs	2
1-1/2 cups	grated raw carrots	375 mL
1 cup	whole wheat flour	250 mL
1/2 cup	all-purpose flour	125 mL
1/2 tsp	baking powder	2 mL
1/2 tsp	baking soda	2 mL
2/3 cup	golden or dark raisins	150 mL
1/2 cup	chopped walnuts or toasted sunflower seeds	125 mL

To toast sunflower seeds: Spread seeds on baking sheet and bake in 350°F (180°C) oven for 5 to 8 minutes, stirring once or twice.

☐ In bowl, cream together butter, brown sugar, vanilla and nutmeg. Add eggs; beat well. Stir in carrots.

☐ Stir together whole wheat and all-purpose flours, baking powder and baking soda. Add to creamed mixture, blending well. Stir in raisins and nuts.

☐ Spread evenly in greased 9-inch (2.5 L) square cake pan. Bake in 350°F (180°C) oven for 35 minutes or until firm to the touch and golden brown. Let cool in pan; cut into 16 squares.

Makes 16 squares.

Calories per square: 196
Grams fat per square: 8.8
Grams fibre per square: 2

Excellent source of: Vitamin A

GLAZED HAZELNUTS AND POPCORN

Preparation time: 10 minutes
Cooking time: 30 minutes

*I*f you plan to serve this snack to children as well as adults, leave out the hot pepper flakes. These nuts are great nibblers for a cocktail party.

2 cups	**hazelnuts (filberts)**	500 mL
4 cups	**popped corn**	1 L
2/3 cup	**granulated sugar**	150 mL
1/4 cup	**water**	50 mL
1 tbsp	**white vinegar**	15 mL
1/4 tsp	**hot pepper sauce**	1 mL
1/4 tsp	**crushed hot pepper flakes (optional)**	1 mL
1/8 tsp	**salt**	0.5 mL
1/8 tsp	**baking soda**	0.5 mL

☐ In shallow baking pan, toast hazelnuts in 325°F (160°C) oven for 5 minutes. Remove from oven. Place in large bowl and mix with popped corn; set aside. Grease baking sheet and set aside.

☐ In small heavy saucepan, stir together sugar, water, vinegar, hot pepper sauce, hot pepper flakes (if using) and salt. Cook over medium-high heat until sugar dissolves and mixture boils.

☐ Reduce heat to medium and place candy thermometer in pot; boil until thermometer registers 310°F (150°C) or until hard-crack stage when a few drops in cold water form hard brittle thread that breaks.

☐ Quickly remove saucepan from heat and stir in baking soda. Pour over hazelnut mixture, stirring to coat evenly. Spread in single layer on prepared pan. Let cool, then break apart. Store in tightly covered container.

Makes about 4 cups (1 L), enough for 8 servings.

Calories per serving: 278
Grams fat per serving: 20.5
Grams fibre per serving: 2

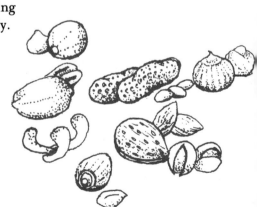

CRISPY ALMOND MIX

Preparation time: 10 minutes
Baking time: 1 hour

T hese easy-to-make nuts are so delicious and intriguing that they'll disappear in no time. You can substitute dry-roasted unsalted peanuts for the almonds.

1	**egg white**	1
1 tsp	**water**	5 mL
2 cups	**almonds (shelled but not blanched)**	500 mL
2 cups	**Shreddies cereal**	500 mL
1/3 cup	**granulated sugar**	75 mL
1 tsp	**cinnamon**	5 mL
1 tsp	**paprika**	5 mL
1/4 tsp	**chili powder**	1 mL

☐ In bowl, beat egg white with water until frothy. Add almonds and Shreddies; stir to coat.

☐ Stir together sugar, cinnamon, paprika and chili powder; add to nuts and toss to coat well.

☐ Spread coated nut mixture in well-greased 13- x 9-inch (3.5 L) baking dish. Bake in 250°F (125°C) oven for 1 hour, stirring every 15 minutes.

Makes 4 cups (1 L), 1/3 cup (75 mL) per serving.

Calories per serving: 189   Good source of: Iron
Grams fat per serving: 12
Grams fibre per serving: 3.9

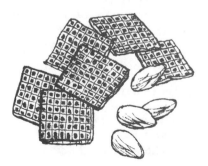

DOUBLE-DECKER DATE BARS

*T*hese treats are simple to make and even easier to eat. Use the blocks of pitted dates found in the baking section of your supermarket, not the tubs of fresh dates in the produce section. Pull dates apart; this way you can check for pits inadvertently left behind.

3/4 lb	**pitted dates, separated**	375 g
1-1/4 cups	**water**	300 mL
1/2 cup	**raisins**	125 mL
33	**graham wafer squares**	33
Frosting:		
1 tbsp	**butter, softened**	15 mL
1 cup	**sifted icing sugar**	250 mL
1/2 tsp	**grated lemon rind**	2 mL
2 to 3 tsp	**lemon juice**	10 to 15 mL

☐ In heavy saucepan, mix together dates, water and raisins; bring to boil. Reduce heat and simmer, stirring occasionally, for 8 minutes or until mixture is thickened but spreadable. Let cool slightly.

☐ Fit 11 graham wafers on bottom of 8-inch (2 L) square cake pan, cutting 2 of them into 3 rectangles each to fit pan snugly. (Use sharp serrated knife to cut wafers with gentle sawing motion.) Gently spread with half of the date mixture.

☐ Press second layer of 11 wafers on top; spread with remaining date mixture. Top with remaining wafers. Refrigerate for 1 hour.

Frosting:
☐ Blend together butter, half of the icing sugar, lemon rind and 1 tsp (5 mL) of the lemon juice. Blend in remaining icing sugar and enough of the remaining lemon juice to make frosting of spreading consistency. Spread over top of wafers. Cut into 18 bars. Cover with plastic wrap or foil and store in refrigerator.

Makes 18 bars.

Calories per bar: 144
Grams fat per bar: 1.9
Grams fibre per bar: 2.6

Notes

over: *Broccoli Dip (page 80) and Chick-Pea Spread (page 81) with*
fresh vegetables and Caraway Crisps (page 143).

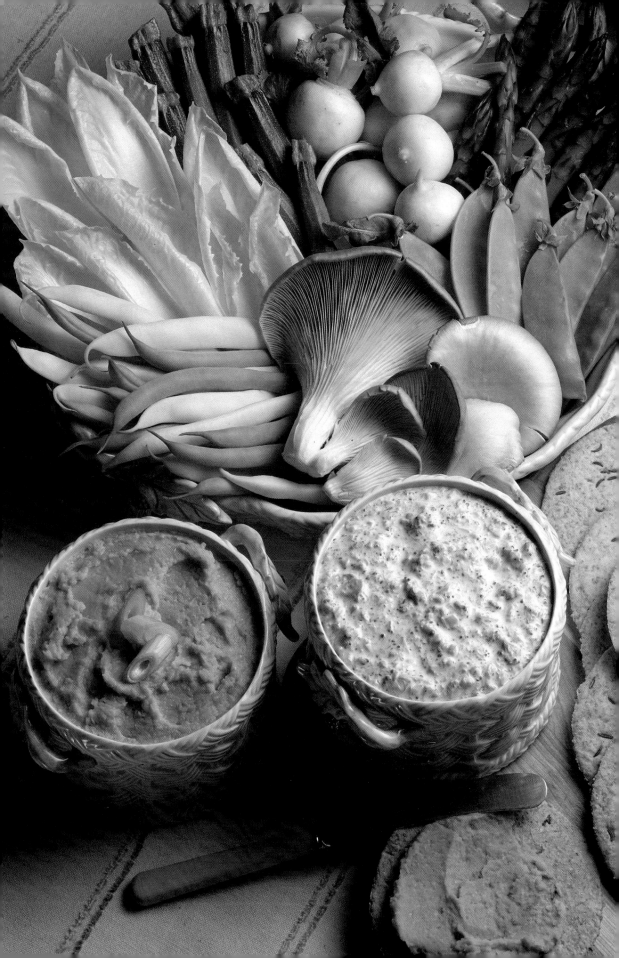

HIGH ENERGY BARS

Preparation time: 20 minutes
Baking time: 35 minutes

Graham flour is a whole-grain wheat flour containing bran. Use it interchangeably with whole wheat flour.

2 cups	graham or whole wheat flour	500 mL
1/2 cup	lightly packed brown sugar	125 mL
1/4 cup	skim milk powder	50 mL
1/4 cup	wheat germ	50 mL
1 tsp	baking powder	5 mL
1 cup	raisins or currants	250 mL
1/2 cup	chopped dried apricots	125 mL
1/2 cup	unsalted sunflower kernels or chopped nuts	125 mL
2	eggs	2
1/2 cup	vegetable oil	125 mL
1/2 cup	molasses	125 mL

Store wheat germ in the refrigerator to prevent its natural oil from becoming rancid.

☐ In large bowl, stir together flour, sugar, skim milk powder, wheat germ and baking powder; stir in raisins, apricots and sunflower kernels.

☐ Mix together eggs, oil and molasses. Add to dry ingredients, blending well. Spread in greased 9-inch (2.5 L) square cake pan.

☐ Bake in 350°F (180°C) oven for 35 minutes or until evenly browned and firm to the touch. Let cool completely and cut into 20 bars.

Makes 20 bars.

Calories per bar: 187 Good source of: Iron
Grams fat per bar: 7.7
Grams fibre per bar: 2.3

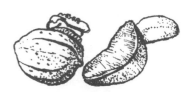

GRANOLA COOKIES

Preparation time: 15 minutes
Baking time: 15 minutes

*F*or the lunch-bag crowd, these cookies are good keepers and travel well.

1/3 cup	**butter**	75 mL
1/3 cup	**packed brown sugar**	75 mL
1/4 cup	**honey**	50 mL
1	**egg**	1
1 tsp	**vanilla**	5 mL
1-1/2 cups	**rolled oats**	375 mL
1/2 cup	**whole wheat flour**	125 mL
1/2 tsp	**salt**	2 mL
1/2 tsp	**cinnamon**	2 mL
1/2 cup	**raisins**	125 mL
1/2 cup	**sunflower seeds**	125 mL
1/2 cup	**sesame seeds**	125 mL
1/2 cup	**desiccated coconut**	125 mL

☐ In large bowl, cream together butter, sugar and honey until light and creamy; beat in egg and vanilla.

☐ Stir together rolled oats, flour, salt and cinnamon; blend into creamed mixture, mixing thoroughly. Add raisins, sunflower seeds, sesame seeds and coconut, stirring well to completely mix.

☐ Drop by rounded teaspoonfuls onto greased baking sheets. Bake in 350°F (180°C) oven for about 15 minutes or until cookies are golden brown.

Makes 2-1/2 dozen cookies.

Calories per cookie: 101
Grams fat per cookie: 5.4
Grams fibre per cookie: 1

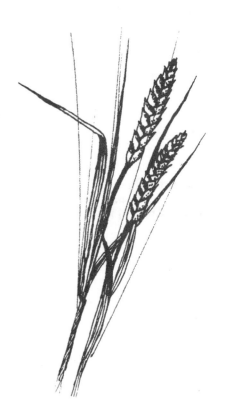

Soups and Salads

Soups can be a great source of fibre, whether a complete meal-in-a-bowl, like a Hearty Bean Soup, or a simple starter like Spinach and Pea Soup. Remember that beans, peas, lentils, avocados and spinach, as well as combinations of vegetables, are high sources of fibre.

Always use a well-flavored stock and, if possible, chill it overnight so that any fat congeals on the surface and can be easily removed. If you use a bouillon cube or powder, or a canned broth, be cautious when adding salt. Always taste first before adjusting seasonings.

To increase the fibre content of a meal planned around soup, try serving one of the high-fibre breads. Caraway Crisps, Onion Casserole Bread, Peppery Corn Bread or Whole Wheat Biscuits all go well with soup.

The high-fibre salads included in this chapter range from whole meal, like Scallop Salad and Warm Chicken Salad with Melon, to simple side salads like Refrigerator Coleslaw. Most salads have fibre, although salads containing beans, peas, avocado, cracked wheat, lentils and the cabbage-related family (brassica vegetables) rate highest. Remember that dressings should be light in oils and eggs to avoid high-fat additions to a healthy meal plan.

HEARTY BEAN CHOWDER

*P*eppery in flavor, this bean and tomato chowder needs only some dark pumpernickel (see page 140) or coarse brown bread and raw vegetable sticks to make a winter supper.

Standing time: 1 hour or overnight
Preparation time: 15 minutes
Cooking time: 1-3/4 hours

1 cup	**dried Great Northern or white pea (navy) beans**	250 mL
1	**stalk celery, cut in chunks**	1
1	**small onion, quartered**	1
1	**bay leaf**	1
1 tbsp	**vegetable oil**	15 mL
2 tsp	**butter**	10 mL
2 cups	**thinly sliced onions**	500 mL
1/4 tsp	**hot pepper flakes**	1 mL
1	**can (28 oz/796 mL) plum tomatoes**	1
1	**sweet green pepper, seeded and sliced**	1
1 tsp	**dried oregano**	5 mL
	Salt	
1/3 lb	**lean ham, diced**	175 g
	Chopped fresh parsley	

☐ Soak beans overnight or by the quick-soak method on page 173; drain.

☐ In heavy saucepan, cover beans with 4 cups (1 L) cold water. Add celery, onion and bay leaf; bring to boil. Reduce heat and simmer, covered, for about 1-1/4 hours or until beans are tender. Drain beans and discard celery, onion and bay leaf; set beans aside.

☐ In same heavy saucepan, heat oil and butter over medium heat. Cook sliced onions and hot pepper flakes, stirring occasionally, for about 10 minutes or until onions are softened and golden but not browned.

☐ Stir in tomatoes, breaking up with wooden spoon; add beans, green pepper, oregano, and salt to taste. Bring to boil; add diced ham. Cover and reduce heat; simmer, stirring occasionally, for 30 minutes. Garnish with chopped parsley.

Makes 8 servings.

Calories per serving: 150
Grams fat per serving: 4.1

Grams fibre per serving: 6
Excellent source of: Vitamin C

Good source of: Vitamin A, iron and thiamine

SPINACH AND PEA SOUP

Thick and satisfying, this soup is full of the flavor of peas. In summer, be sure to use fresh peas. For a thinner soup, add 1 cup (250 mL) milk.

1 tbsp	butter	15 mL
2	leeks (white parts only), sliced	2
2 cups	frozen peas	500 mL
2 cups	torn fresh spinach, packed	500 mL
2 cups	chicken stock	500 mL
1/4 tsp	dried savory	1 mL
	Salt and freshly ground pepper	
	Plain yogurt	

To make a designer swirl with yogurt: Drizzle yogurt onto soup in a back and forth pattern. Draw a skewer or toothpick back and forth through yogurt in opposite direction to make a zigzag pattern.

☐ In saucepan, melt butter over medium heat; cook leeks until soft and fragrant but not browned.

☐ Add peas, spinach, chicken stock and savory. Bring to boil; reduce heat, cover and simmer for 20 minutes.

☐ In food processor or blender, purée soup, in batches, until smooth. Season with salt and pepper to taste. Serve with a drizzle of yogurt on top of each serving.

Makes 4 servings.

Calories per serving: 118
Grams fat per serving: 3.8
Grams fibre per serving: 9.1

Excellent source of: Vitamin A
Good source of: Iron, niacin
   and vitamin C

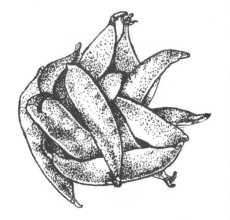

MIX-AND-MATCH VEGETABLE SOUP

Preparation time: 15 minutes
Cooking time: 20 to 25 minutes

*T*o vary the flavor, you can change the vegetables each time you make this chunky and light soup. Substitute two sliced leeks for the onion, watercress for the parsley, 1-1/2 cups (375 mL) diced rutabaga for the carrots, and peas and celery for the cabbage.

4 cups	chicken stock	1 L
1	medium onion, quartered	1
1/4 cup	chopped fresh parsley	50 mL
1/4 cup	chopped fresh dill	50 mL
2	carrots, sliced	2
2	large potatoes, cubed	2
1	bay leaf	1
6 cups	torn fresh spinach, packed	1.5 L
2 cups	shredded cabbage	500 mL
	Salt and freshly ground pepper	
	Croutons	

To make 2 cups (500 mL) croutons: Remove crusts from 4 slices of day-old bread, preferably whole wheat. Lightly butter slices and cut into cubes. Spread on ungreased baking sheet and bake in 400°F (200°C) oven for about 5 minutes or until evenly browned, turning once.

☐ In large saucepan, bring chicken stock to boil; add onion, parsley, dill, carrots, potatoes and bay leaf. Simmer, covered, until potatoes are tender, about 15 minutes. Remove bay leaf.

☐ Add spinach and cabbage; cook, covered, for 5 to 7 minutes or until cabbage is softened. Season with salt and pepper to taste. Serve with croutons.

Makes 6 servings.

Calories per serving: 99
Grams fat per serving: 1.2
Grams fibre per serving: 5.6

Excellent source of: Vitamins A and C
Good source of: Iron and niacin

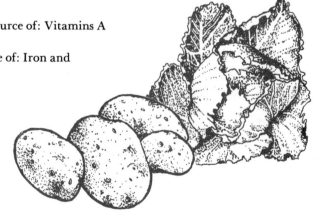

SPLIT PEA SOUP

Preparation time: 15 minutes
Cooking time: 1 hour

A full-bodied soup, this makes a complete light supper when teamed with brown bread and a green salad.

1 tbsp	**vegetable oil**	15 mL
1 cup	**chopped carrots**	250 mL
1 cup	**chopped celery**	250 mL
2	**leeks, sliced**	2
1	**clove garlic, chopped**	1
3 cups	**chicken stock**	750 mL
3 cups	**water**	750 mL
1-1/2 cups	**split yellow peas**	375 mL
1/2 tsp	**salt**	2 mL
1/4 tsp	**dried thyme**	1 mL
Dash	**hot pepper sauce**	Dash

☐ In large saucepan, heat oil over medium heat; cook carrots, celery, leeks and garlic for about 5 minutes or until softened and fragrant. Do not brown.

☐ Stir in chicken stock, water, split peas, salt, thyme and hot pepper sauce; bring to boil. Cover and reduce heat to low; simmer, stirring occasionally, for about 1 hour or until peas are tender.

Makes 6 servings.

Calories per serving: 106
Grams fat per serving: 3
Grams fibre per serving: 3.1

Excellent source of: Vitamin A

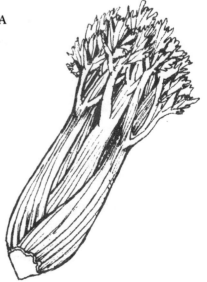

PEASANT SOUP WITH PESTO

Preparation time: 1 hour or overnight
Cooking time: 1 hour and 10 minutes

*T*his hearty peasant-style soup from France has pesto, or *pistou* in French, swirled into it. You can reduce the fat in this recipe by serving the soup without pesto.

Soup:

1-1/2 cups	white pea (navy) beans	375 mL
2 tbsp	olive oil	25 mL
3	onions, chopped (about 1 cup/250 mL)	3
1 cup	chopped celery	250 mL
3	carrots, sliced (about 1-1/2 cups/375 mL)	3
3	small zucchini, unpeeled and sliced (about 1-1/2 cups/375 mL)	3
8 cups	water (half chicken stock, if desired)	2 L
2	bay leaves	2
1 tsp	salt	5 mL
1/4 tsp	dried savory	1 mL
	Freshly ground pepper	
2 cups	frozen lima beans (12 oz/350 g package)	500 mL

Pesto:

2 cups	fresh basil leaves	500 mL
3	cloves garlic, minced	3
2/3 cup	freshly grated Parmesan or Romano cheese	150 mL
1/4 cup	pine nuts, toasted	50 mL
1/4 cup	olive oil	50 mL

To toast pine nuts: Stir-cook nuts in an ungreased small skillet over medium-high heat until lightly browned.

If fresh basil is unavailable for pesto, use 2 cups (500 mL) fresh parsley leaves and 2 tsp (10 mL) dried basil. It will not be quite the same flavor, but will still be delicious.

Soup:

☐ Soak beans overnight or by the quick-soak method on page 173; drain.

☐ In large heavy saucepan or Dutch oven, heat oil over medium heat; cook onions and celery, stirring, for 5 minutes. Add carrots and zucchini; cook, stirring, for 5 minutes. With slotted spoon, remove vegetables and set aside.

☐ Pour water into pan and bring to boil; add beans, bay leaves, salt, savory, and pepper to taste. Simmer, partially covered, for 40 minutes. Return vegetable mixture to pan along with lima beans; simmer, partially covered, for 30 minutes or until beans are tender. Remove bay leaves. Taste and adjust seasoning.

Pesto:
☐ Rinse and dry basil; shred with French knife or kitchen shears. In blender or food processor, combine basil, garlic, cheese, pine nuts and oil; process, using on/off motion, until smooth, scraping down sides of container often.

☐ To serve, ladle soup into tureen and swirl in pesto; alternatively, add a spoonful to each serving.

Makes 8 servings.

Calories per serving: 327
Grams fat per serving: 16
Grams fibre per serving: 9.6

Excellent source of: Vitamin A
Good source of: Calcium, phosphorus, iron and vitamin C

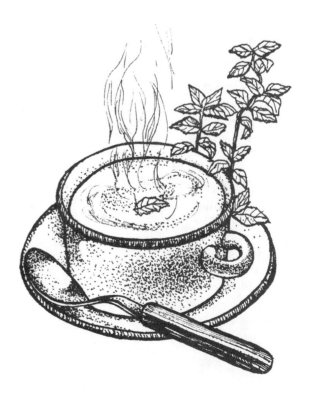

GREENS AND FRUIT WITH CURRY VINAIGRETTE

Preparation time: 10 minutes

Give this salad a special touch by serving it on thin slices of peeled avocado. Brush the cut surfaces of the avocado with lemon juice to prevent browning.

2 cups	torn romaine lettuce	500 mL
2 cups	torn fresh spinach	500 mL
2	oranges, peeled and sliced	2
1/2 cup	red or green seedless grapes, halved	125 mL
1/4 cup	toasted sliced almonds	50 mL
Curry Vinaigrette:		
2 tbsp	vegetable oil	25 mL
2 tbsp	white wine vinegar	25 mL
2 tbsp	finely chopped fresh chives	25 mL
1 tbsp	packed brown sugar	15 mL
1 tsp	(approx) curry powder	5 mL
1/2 tsp	soy sauce	2 mL

To toast almonds: Spread on baking sheet and bake in 350°F (180°C) oven for 5 minutes or until golden.

Avocados are a good source of fibre but they are also very high in fat, so use them only occasionally.

☐ In large bowl, combine lettuce, spinach, orange slices, grapes and almonds. Refrigerate until serving time.

Curry Vinaigrette:
☐ In small bowl, blend together oil, vinegar, chives, sugar, curry powder and soy sauce, adding more curry to taste, if desired.

☐ Just before serving, whisk dressing until blended; pour over salad and toss to coat lightly.

Makes 8 servings.

Calories per serving: 92
Grams fat per serving: 6.1
Grams fibre per serving: 2.1

Excellent source of: Vitamins A and C

CHUTNEY RICE SALAD

*F*or individual servings of this intriguing salad, pack into six lightly greased custard cups. Cover with plastic or foil wrap and refrigerate overnight. At serving time, turn them out onto salad greens.

3 cups	**cooked brown rice, chilled** (3/4 cup/175 mL uncooked)	750 mL
1-1/4 cups	**finely chopped unpeeled Granny Smith apples**	300 mL
1 cup	**thinly sliced celery**	250 mL
1/2 cup	**golden raisins**	125 mL
1/2 cup	Mango Chutney (see recipe page 172)	125 mL
1/4 cup	**toasted slivered almonds**	50 mL
1/4 cup	**vegetable oil**	50 mL
	Lettuce	

☐ In large bowl, combine rice, apples, celery, raisins, chutney, almonds and oil; chill for about 15 minutes for flavors to blend.

☐ Serve in lettuce cups or on bed of shredded lettuce.

Makes 6 servings.

Calories per serving: 351
Grams fat per serving: 15.8
Grams fibre per serving: 2.7

Good source of: Phosphorus, iron, vitamins A and C

To cook long-grain brown rice: Add brown rice to three times its volume of boiling water (salted if desired). Cover, reduce heat to low and cook for 45 minutes or until rice is tender and water has been absorbed. Let stand for 5 minutes, then fluff with a fork.

Because brown rice has the bran layer, or coating, left on, it should be stored in the refrigerator for up to 6 months. This will prevent the oils left in the germ of the rice grains from becoming rancid.

To toast slivered almonds: Spread on baking sheet and bake in 350°F (180°C) oven for 5 minutes or until golden.

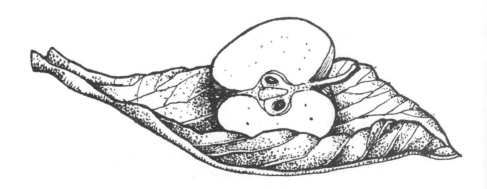

WARM CHICKEN SALAD WITH MELON

Preparation time: 15 minutes
Cooking time: 5 minutes

*A*n edible flower (such as a daisy or nasturtium) adds a summery garnish to this salad. In fall, sprinkle it with pomegranate seeds, and in winter, brighten the dish with snipped fresh parsley.

1	whole chicken breast, skinned and boned	1
1 tbsp	vegetable oil	15 mL
1/3 cup	white wine vinegar or rice wine vinegar	75 mL
3 tbsp	granulated sugar	50 mL
2 tbsp	lime juice	25 mL
2 tbsp	light soy sauce	25 mL
2 tsp	cornstarch	10 mL
1 tsp	grated lime rind	5 mL
Dash	hot pepper sauce	Dash
1	small cantaloupe, cut in balls or chunks	1
2	oranges, sectioned	2
4 cups	torn mixed salad greens (romaine, spinach, endive)	1 L

☐ Cut chicken across the grain into 1/4-inch (5 mm) strips. Heat large skillet or wok over high heat until hot; add oil and heat until hot but not smoking. Add chicken and stir-fry until meat turns white, 3 to 4 minutes. Remove and set aside.

☐ Mix together vinegar, sugar, lime juice, soy sauce, cornstarch, lime rind and hot pepper sauce. Add to skillet, stirring until mixture boils. Remove from heat.

☐ Return chicken to skillet along with cantaloupe and orange sections; toss lightly to coat with sauce. Spoon over greens in salad bowl. Serve at once.

Makes 4 servings.

Calories per serving: 241
Grams fat per serving: 5.8
Grams fibre per serving: 4.2

Excellent source of: Vitamins A and C and niacin
Good source of: Iron and phosphorus

JELLIED GAZPACHO

*S*erve this with a drizzle of yogurt and a sprinkle of snipped fresh chives.

2	envelopes unflavored gelatin	2
2-1/2 cups	tomato or vegetable juice	625 mL
2 tbsp	wine vinegar	25 mL
1 tbsp	packed brown sugar	15 mL
1 tsp	salt	5 mL
1 tsp	Worcestershire sauce	5 mL
Dash	hot pepper sauce	Dash
2	tomatoes, diced	2
1 cup	chopped unpeeled cucumber	250 mL
1/2 cup	diced sweet green pepper	125 mL
1/4 cup	chopped green onion	50 mL
3 cups	shredded fresh spinach	750 mL

Use your microwave oven to dissolve the gelatin for Jellied Gazpacho. Sprinkle gelatin over 1/2 cup (125 mL) tomato juice and let stand for 5 minutes. Microwave at Medium (50% power) for 1 to 1-1/2 minutes or until gelatin has dissolved.

☐ In saucepan over low heat, sprinkle gelatin over 1/2 cup (125 mL) of the tomato juice; heat until gelatin has dissolved. Remove from heat and add remaining 2 cups (500 mL) juice, vinegar, sugar, salt, Worcestershire and hot pepper sauce. Chill until slightly thickened but not set (the consistency of unbeaten egg whites).

☐ Meanwhile, mix together tomatoes, cucumber, green pepper and onion. Fold into chilled gelatin mixture. Pour into rinsed 6-cup (1.5 L) mould. Chill until firm.

☐ To serve, unmould onto bed of spinach.

Makes 6 servings.

Calories per serving: 53
Grams fat per serving: 0.3
Grams fibre per serving: 2

Excellent source of: Vitamins
A and C

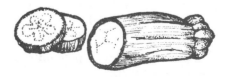

MOCK PASTA SALAD

Baking time: 1 hour
Preparation time: 15 minutes
Chilling time: 1 hour

*I*f you have a large spaghetti squash, cook as directed and serve half as a hot vegetable for supper. Remove the spaghetti-like strands of the remaining half and chill overnight to use in this salad.

Salad:

1	small spaghetti squash	1
4 cups	torn fresh spinach, packed	1 L
1-1/2 cups	sliced mushrooms	375 mL
1 cup	cherry tomatoes, halved	250 mL
3	green onions, diagonally sliced	3

Basil Vinaigrette:

1/3 cup	vegetable oil	75 mL
1/4 cup	tomato juice	50 mL
2 tbsp	white wine vinegar	25 mL
2 tbsp	chopped fresh basil or 2 tsp (10 mL) dried	25 mL
1 tbsp	chopped fresh oregano or 1 tsp (5 mL) dried	15 mL
1 tbsp	Dijon mustard	15 mL
1	clove garlic, minced	1
	Freshly ground pepper	

Garnish:

1/4 cup	pine nuts, toasted	50 mL
2 tbsp	freshly grated Parmesan cheese	25 mL

To toast pine nuts: Stir-cook nuts in an ungreased small skillet over medium-high heat until lightly browned.

☐ Bake squash in 350°F (180°C) oven for 1 hour or until tender when pierced with fork. Let cool to room temperature. Cut in half; remove seeds. With fork, remove spaghetti-like strands. Place strands in large serving bowl; cover and refrigerate until thoroughly chilled.

☐ Add spinach to chilled squash along with mushrooms, tomatoes and onions; toss lightly.

Basil Vinaigrette:
☐ In blender or bowl, combine oil, tomato juice, vinegar, basil, oregano, mustard, garlic, and pepper to taste; process or beat with wire whisk until well blended. Pour over salad and toss lightly.

Garnish:
☐ Sprinkle salad with pine nuts; dust lightly with cheese. Serve immediately.

Makes 6 servings.

Calories per serving: 200
Grams fat per serving: 15.8
Grams fibre per serving: 4.3

Excellent source of: Vitamins
A and C
Good source of: Iron

PASTA NIÇOISE

Preparation time: 15 minutes
Chilling time: 2 hours

*T*his pasta makes an easy dish to carry to a potluck party, and is just right for a backyard supper.

1/2 lb	**pasta (shells, fusilli, penne, rotini)**	250 g
1/2 lb	**green beans, sliced**	250 g
1	**can (6.5 oz/184 g) flaked tuna, packed in broth**	1
1 cup	**cherry tomatoes, halved**	250 mL
1 cup	**sliced celery**	250 mL
1/4 cup	**chopped green onion**	50 mL
1/2 cup	**sliced black olives**	125 mL
1	**clove garlic, chopped**	1
1/4 cup	**chopped fresh parsley**	50 mL
3 tbsp	**olive oil**	50 mL
2 tbsp	**lemon juice**	25 mL
2 tbsp	**white wine vinegar**	25 mL
1/2 tsp	**salt**	2 mL
	Freshly ground pepper	

☐ Cook pasta according to package directions or until *al dente* (tender but firm). Drain and rinse under cold water; drain again. Steam green beans for 5 minutes; refresh under cold water to stop cooking.

☐ Drain tuna; toss together with pasta, green beans, tomatoes, celery, onion and olives. In small bowl, mix together garlic, parsley, oil, lemon juice, vinegar, salt, and pepper to taste; stir well. Pour over salad; toss to coat. Refrigerate for at least 2 hours.

Makes 6 servings.

Calories per serving: 283
Grams fat per serving: 8.6
Grams fibre per serving: 3.4

Excellent source of: Vitamin C
and niacin
Good source of: Phosphorus,
iron, vitamin A and thiamine

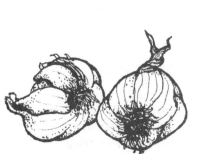

SCALLOP SALAD

Chilling time: 1 hour
Preparation time: 15 minutes

*T*his easy dish makes a wonderful luncheon or supper salad for any occasion. Prepare the scallops early in the day, then toss the salad together just before serving in lettuce cups or spooned over thin melon wedges.

2 cups	water	500 mL
2 tbsp	lemon juice	25 mL
2	slices onion	2
1/2 tsp	salt	2 mL
1 lb	scallops, thawed if frozen	500 g
1 cup	grapefruit sections	250 mL
1/2 cup	sliced celery	125 mL
8	stuffed olives, sliced	8
1	large firm banana, sliced	1
1	small apple, unpeeled, cored and sliced	1
Dressing:		
1/4 cup	mayonnaise	50 mL
1 tbsp	grapefruit juice	15 mL
1 tsp	lemon juice	5 mL
1/4 tsp	salt	1 mL
1/4 tsp	curry powder	1 mL

☐ In saucepan, bring water, lemon juice, onion and salt to boil; add scallops. Reduce heat, cover and simmer for 2 to 3 minutes or until centre of scallop is opaque and white. (Do not overcook or scallops will be tough.) Drain and refrigerate scallops until chilled.

☐ In bowl, combine scallops, grapefruit, celery, olives, banana and apple.

Dressing:
☐ Blend together mayonnaise, grapefruit and lemon juices, salt and curry powder; pour over salad and toss lightly.

Makes 6 servings.

Calories per serving: 161
Grams fat per serving: 6.1
Grams fibre per serving: 2.5

Excellent source of: Vitamin C

Notes

over: *Spinach and Pea Soup (page 93) and Onion Casserole Bread (page 142).*

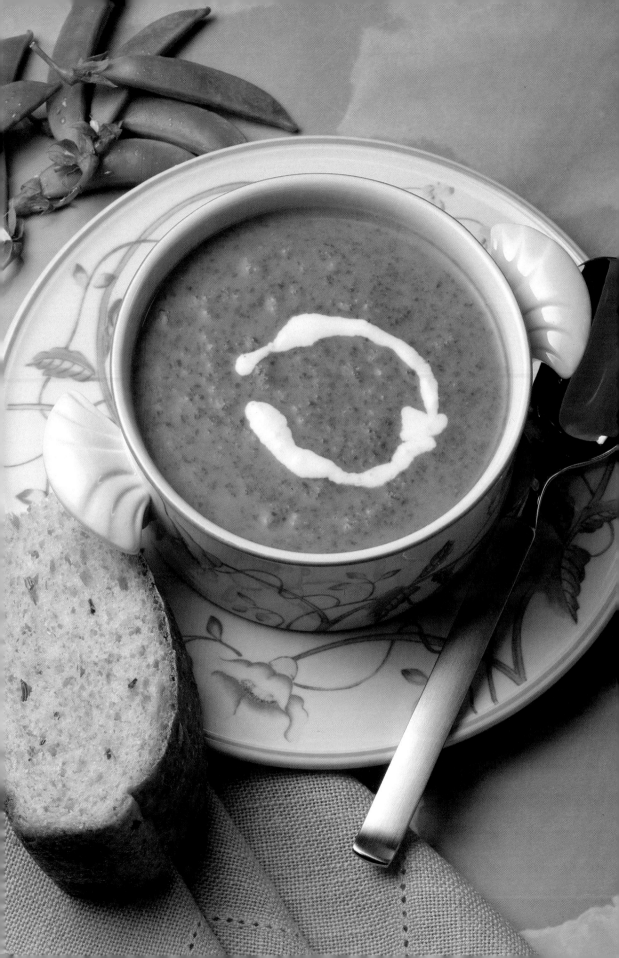

REFRIGERATOR COLESLAW

Preparation time: 15 minutes
Chilling time: 4 hours or
overnight

*F*or an impressive serving dish, hollow out a well-shaped green cabbage and spoon the chilled slaw into the cabbage "bowl". Use the inside leaves to make this salad.

4 cups	**shredded cabbage**	1 L
1/2 cup	**chopped celery**	125 mL
1/2 cup	**chopped Spanish onion**	125 mL
1	**small sweet green pepper, slivered**	1
2	**carrots, grated**	2
Dressing:		
1/3 cup	**white vinegar**	75 mL
1/4 cup	**vegetable oil**	50 mL
1/3 cup	**granulated sugar**	75 mL
1 tsp	**celery seed**	5 mL
1 tsp	**salt**	5 mL
1/2 tsp	**freshly ground pepper**	2 mL
1/2 tsp	**dry mustard**	2 mL

☐ In large bowl, combine cabbage, celery, onion, green pepper and carrots.

Dressing:
☐ In small saucepan, combine vinegar, oil, sugar, celery seed, salt, pepper and mustard; bring to full boil, stirring until sugar dissolves. Pour over cabbage mixture. Refrigerate, covered, for at least 4 hours or overnight.

☐ At serving time, toss lightly to mix well.

Makes 8 servings.

Calories per serving: 117
Grams fat per serving: 6.8
Grams fibre per serving: 2.5

Excellent source of: Vitamins
  A and C

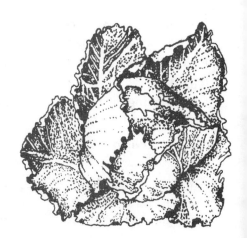

CRACKED WHEAT SALAD

Preparation time: 50 minutes
Chilling time: 1 hour

*T*he busy hostess will appreciate this delicious salad, sometimes called tabbouleh, because it can be prepared a day ahead of time. Serve it in lettuce cups for an attractive presentation. It's also perfect for carrying to a picnic, but pack the yogurt and mint separately and add them to the salad at the picnic site. If fresh mint is unavailable, use chopped fresh parsley for color.

1 cup	**cracked wheat (bulgur)**	250 mL
1	**can (19 oz/540 mL) chick-peas, drained**	1
1 cup	**shredded carrots**	250 mL
1 cup	**cooked sliced green beans**	250 mL
2	**tomatoes, cut in wedges**	2
1 cup	**sliced mushrooms**	250 mL
1/2 cup	**sliced green onions**	125 mL
3 tbsp	**vegetable oil**	50 mL
3 tbsp	**lemon juice**	50 mL
1 tsp	**salt**	5 mL
1/2 tsp	**granulated sugar**	2 mL
	Freshly ground pepper	
Topping:		
1 cup	**plain yogurt**	250 mL
2 tbsp	**chopped fresh mint**	25 mL

Bulgur is a form of cracked wheat that has already been steamed and dried. Use either a fine or medium grind for Cracked Wheat Salad.

☐ In large bowl, cover cracked wheat with 2 cups (500 mL) boiling water. Let stand for 45 minutes; drain well.

☐ Add chick-peas, carrots, green beans, tomatoes, mushrooms, green onions, oil, lemon juice, salt, sugar, and pepper to taste; toss well. Chill for at least 1 hour.

Topping:
☐ At serving time, mix together yogurt and mint; spoon over each serving.

Makes 8 servings.

Calories per serving: 220
Grams fat per serving: 6.7
Grams fibre per serving: 5.7

Excellent source of: Vitamin A
Good source of: Phosphorus, iron and vitamin C

Main Courses, Vegetables and Side Dishes

Since meat, fish, poultry, eggs and cheese by themselves contain little fibre, vegetables, dried fruits, seeds and dried beans are added to our recipes to give fibre-rich main dishes. If eating plain meats appeals to you, be sure to choose from the vegetable and side dishes in this chapter to increase your fibre intake. Consulting the chart on page 5 will help you choose vegetables for added fibre.

Today's food styles include stir-fry cooking Chinese-style, Mexican foods loaded with beans, corn and guacamole, Italian pastas with an endless variety of sauces and toppings including vegetables and nuts, and Thai spring rolls filled with combinations of vegetables. If ethnic cooking is not for you, our Canadian heritage boasts French-Canadian pea soup, hearty western baked beans, good-for-the-soul peasant stews with lots of potatoes and other root vegetables, cabbage rolls, meat loaf and chili. All these dishes are good sources of fibre.

As well, side dishes with lentils, barley, bulgur (cracked wheat) and any of the pulses (beans, peas, legumes) make great additions to the meal.

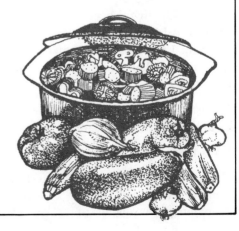

STIR-FRIED BEEF AND CHINESE CABBAGE

Marinating time: 3 hours
Preparation time: 20 minutes
Cooking time: 10 minutes

Stir-fry suppers are especially quick to make when you plan ahead. Be sure to have all the vegetables sliced before you start and allow enough time for the beef to marinate.

2 tbsp	**vegetable oil**	25 mL
1 tbsp	**soy sauce**	15 mL
1 tbsp	**rice wine vinegar**	15 mL
1 tbsp	**cornstarch**	15 mL
1 tsp	**granulated sugar**	5 mL
1/2 tsp	**salt**	2 mL
1/2 lb	**flank steak, thinly sliced**	250 g
4 cups	**shredded Chinese cabbage**	1 L
1 cup	**sliced celery**	250 mL
1/2 cup	**sliced green onions**	125 mL
1 tbsp	**finely chopped gingerroot**	15 mL
1/4 cup	**chicken stock**	50 mL
3 cups	**hot cooked rice**	750 mL
	Toasted sesame seeds (optional)	

To toast sesame seeds: Stir-cook seeds in ungreased skillet over medium-high heat until lightly browned.

☐ In plastic bag set in bowl, combine 1 tbsp (15 mL) of the oil, soy sauce, vinegar, 1 tsp (5 mL) of the cornstarch, sugar and salt. Add flank steak slices. Seal bag and marinate in refrigerator overnight, or at room temperature for 2 to 3 hours, turning bag frequently.

☐ When ready to cook, remove meat slices. Add remaining cornstarch to marinade and set aside.

☐ In wok or large skillet, heat remaining oil over high heat. Quickly stir-fry beef for 2 to 3 minutes or until browned. Add cabbage, celery, onions and gingerroot; stir-fry for 1 minute. Stir in chicken stock; cover and cook for 3 minutes. Pour in reserved marinade; cook, stirring, just until sauce is clear and thickened.

☐ Taste and adjust seasoning if necessary. Serve over hot rice and sprinkle with sesame seeds, if using.

Makes 4 servings.

Calories per serving: 329
Grams fat per serving: 10.9
Grams fibre per serving: 3.7

Excellent source of: Vitamins A and C, niacin and iron
Good source of: Phosphorus

CRANBURGERS

Preparation time: 10 minutes
Cooking time: 5 to 10 minutes

*C*hopped fresh or frozen cranberries add moisture and color to ordinary burgers. They're delicious when accompanied with lettuce, mustard and sliced sweet pickles or relish. Serve on whole wheat buns, if available.

1-1/2 lb	**lean ground beef**	750 g
1 cup	**cranberries, chopped**	250 mL
1/4 cup	**finely chopped onion**	50 mL
1 tbsp	**packed brown sugar**	15 mL
1 tsp	**salt**	5 mL
1 tsp	**Worcestershire sauce**	5 mL
	Freshly ground pepper	
1	**egg**	1

☐ In bowl, combine beef, cranberries, onion, sugar, salt, Worcestershire sauce, pepper to taste and egg; mix lightly. Shape into 6 patties.

☐ Broil or barbecue patties to desired doneness. Serve at once.

Makes 6 servings.

Calories per serving: 341
Grams fat per serving: 13
Grams fibre per serving: 2

Excellent source of: Iron and niacin
Good source of: Phosphorus and thiamine

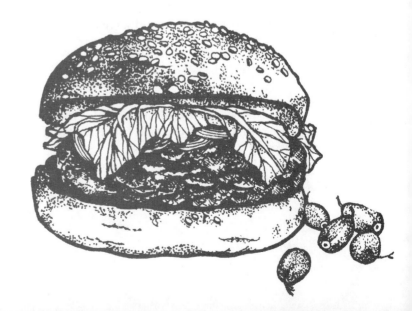

PASTA WITH SPINACH PESTO

Preparation time: 10 minutes
Cooking time: 10 minutes

*L*overs of Italian food will be familiar with flavorful basil pesto, but you'll love this spinach version with its extra flavor and fibre. Whole wheat pasta (fresh or dry packaged) will add even more fibre plus a fabulous flavor variation you will enjoy.

1/2 lb	spaghettini	250 g
Spinach Pesto:		
1/4 cup	pine nuts, toasted	50 mL
1 or 2	cloves garlic	1 or 2
2 cups	fresh spinach, packed	500 mL
1/4 cup	freshly grated Parmesan or Romano cheese	50 mL
3 tbsp	olive oil	50 mL
1/2 tsp	salt	2 mL
	Freshly ground pepper	

To toast pine nuts: Stir-cook nuts in an ungreased small skillet over medium-high heat until lightly browned.

☐ In large pot of rapidly boiling water, cook spaghettini according to package directions or until *al dente* (tender but firm).

Spinach Pesto:
☐ Meanwhile, in food processor or blender, process nuts until finely ground. Add garlic and spinach; process until finely chopped. Add cheese, oil, salt, and pepper to taste; process until well blended.

☐ Drain spaghettini; toss with pesto and serve immediately.

Makes 4 servings.

Calories per serving: 342
Grams fat per serving: 16.8
Grams fibre per serving: 2.4

Excellent source of: Vitamin A
Good source of: Phosphorus and iron

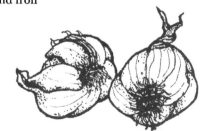

ROTINI WITH PEAS AND PROSCIUTTO

Preparation time: 15 minutes
Cooking time: 15 minutes

*R*otini is a pasta shaped like corkscrews. You can use fusilli, medium shells or penne instead. If prosciutto is unavailable, substitute ham or bacon.

4	slices prosciutto, chopped	4
2	cloves garlic, chopped	2
1	medium onion, chopped	1
1 cup	chopped tomatoes	250 mL
1 cup	fresh or frozen peas	250 mL
1/2 cup	chicken stock	125 mL
1/4 cup	red wine	50 mL
2 tbsp	tomato paste	25 mL
1/4 tsp	dried basil	1 mL
1/4 tsp	hot pepper flakes	1 mL
	Salt and freshly ground pepper	
1/2 lb	rotini	250 g
2 tbsp	chopped fresh parsley	25 mL
	Freshly grated Romano or Parmesan cheese	

☐ In large skillet over medium heat, sauté prosciutto with garlic and onion until onion is softened. Add tomatoes, peas, chicken stock, red wine, tomato paste, basil, hot pepper flakes, and salt and pepper to taste. Simmer, uncovered, for 15 minutes.

☐ Meanwhile, in saucepan of boiling salted water, cook pasta according to package directions or until *al dente* (tender but firm). Drain and transfer to serving dish. Pour sauce over top. Sprinkle with chopped parsley. Add cheese to taste.

Makes 6 servings.

Calories per serving: 216
Grams fat per serving: 3.9
Grams fibre per serving: 4

Excellent source of: Vitamin C
Good source of: Vitamin A, thiamine, iron, phosphorus and niacin

STEAK AND KIDNEY STEW WITH WHOLE WHEAT DUMPLINGS

Preparation time: 20 minutes
Cooking time: 1 hour

One of the old-fashioned "comfort foods", this stew is topped with whole wheat dumplings. If you prefer, you can top the stew with Whole Wheat Biscuits (see recipe, page 139) after the meat has simmered. Just arrange the unbaked biscuits on top of the stew and bake in 425°F (220°C) oven for 18 to 20 minutes or until biscuits are browned.

3/4 lb	round steak	375 g
3/4 lb	kidneys	375 g
1	large onion, chopped	1
1-1/2 cups	beef stock	375 mL
1 tbsp	Worcestershire sauce	15 mL
1/2 tsp	salt	2 mL
1/2 tsp	dried savory OR 1/4 tsp (1 mL) each dried thyme and oregano	2 mL
	Freshly ground pepper	
3 tbsp	all-purpose flour	50 mL
1-1/2 cups	peas, fresh or frozen	375 mL
Whole Wheat Dumplings:		
1/2 cup	whole wheat flour	125 mL
1/2 cup	all-purpose flour	125 mL
1 tsp	baking powder	5 mL
1/2 tsp	baking soda	2 mL
1/4 tsp	salt	1 mL
1	egg	1
1/2 cup	buttermilk	125 mL
2 tbsp	vegetable oil	25 mL
2 tbsp	chopped fresh parsley	25 mL

☐ Trim visible fat from steak; cut into 3/4-inch (2 cm) cubes. Trim kidneys; cut into 1/2-inch (1 cm) pieces.

☐ In large skillet over medium heat, combine steak cubes, kidneys, onion, beef stock, Worcestershire sauce, salt, savory, and pepper to taste. Cover and simmer until meat is tender, about 45 minutes. Taste and adjust seasoning.

☐ Mix 3 tbsp (50 mL) flour with 1/4 cup (50 mL) cold water. Add to meat mixture and cook over medium heat, stirring constantly, until thickened. Add peas.

Whole Wheat Dumpings:
☐ In bowl, mix together whole wheat and all-purpose flours, baking powder, baking soda and salt. In separate bowl, blend egg with buttermilk and oil; add to flour mixture, stirring just to blend.

☐ Drop spoonfuls of dumpling batter evenly over top of stew. Sprinkle with parsley. Cover and simmer for about 15 minutes or until dumplings feel firm and cake tester inserted in centre comes out clean.

Makes 6 servings.

Calories per serving: 342
Grams fat per serving: 14.8
Grams fibre per serving: 4.4

Excellent source of: Iron, riboflavin and niacin
Good source of: Vitamins A and C, thiamine and phosphorus

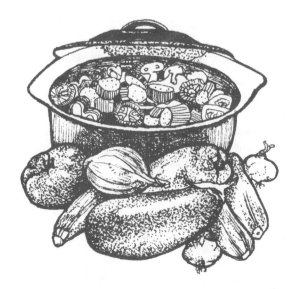

MOUSSAKA

Preparation time: 15 minutes
Baking time: 20 minutes

Be sure to use a low-fat or partly skimmed milk cheese to reduce fat in this light version of a typical Greek dish.

1	**medium onion, chopped**	1
1 tbsp	**olive oil**	15 mL
1 lb	**lean ground beef or lamb**	500 g
1	**can (14 oz/398 mL) tomato sauce**	1
1/2 cup	**dry red wine or beef stock**	125 mL
1/2 tsp	**dried thyme**	2 mL
1/4 tsp	**cinnamon**	1 mL
1	**eggplant, about 1-1/2 lb (750 g), sliced and baked**	1
1-1/2 cups	**shredded Monterey Jack or mozzarella cheese**	375 mL
2 tbsp	**chopped fresh parsley**	25 mL

☐ In large skillet, cook onion in oil over medium heat for about 5 minutes or until onion is softened but not browned. Add beef; cook, stirring often, until crumbly and no longer pink.

☐ Stir in tomato sauce, wine, thyme and cinnamon; simmer, uncovered, for 10 minutes, stirring occasionally.

☐ In shallow 11- x 7-inch (2 L) baking dish or casserole, arrange half of the baked eggplant slices. Top with meat mixture, then remaining eggplant. Sprinkle with cheese and parsley. Bake in 375°F (190°C) oven for about 20 minutes or until bubbly and golden.

Makes 6 servings.

Calories per serving: 328
Grams fat per serving: 15.8
Grams fibre per serving: 2.9

Excellent source of: Phosphorus
 and niacin
Good source of: Calcium, iron,
 vitamins A and C

Often we pass up eggplant because it soaks up too much fat while cooking. To make baked eggplant slices, salt the cut surfaces and let the slices drain in a colander for 30 minutes to reduce the amount of oil absorbed in cooking. Be sure to rinse off the salt under cold water; drain on paper towels and pat dry.

Lightly brush the slices with oil and bake in a single layer in a 425°F (220°C) oven until lightly browned and tender. Prepare them this way for recipes calling for browned, sautéed eggplant slices, such as Moussaka. Depending on their size and ripeness, slices will take 20 to 35 minutes to cook. Turn occasionally for even browning. Sprinkle with about 2 tsp (10 mL) dry herbs, such as basil, oregano, rosemary or thyme for extra flavor. Minced garlic can be sprinkled over top of slices before baking.

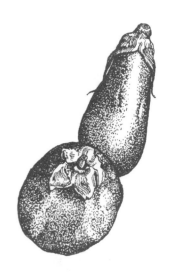

LIMA BEAN BAKE

A change from ordinary baked beans, this dish has a delicious chili flavor.

Soaking time: 1 hour or
overnight
Preparation time: 20 minutes
Baking time: 1 hour

1-1/2 cups	**dry lima beans**	375 mL
1/2 tsp	**salt**	2 mL
1	**can (19 oz/540 mL) tomatoes, undrained**	1
1 cup	**chopped onion**	250 mL
1	**clove garlic, minced**	1
1/4 cup	**cider vinegar**	50 mL
1 tbsp	**molasses**	15 mL
2 tsp	**chili powder**	10 mL
2 tsp	**Worcestershire sauce**	10 mL

☐ Soak beans overnight or by the quick-soak method on page 173. Bring beans in their soaking liquid to boil and add salt; cook for about 15 minutes or just until beans are tender.

☐ Drain beans and stir in tomatoes, onion, garlic, vinegar, molasses, chili powder and Worcestershire sauce; mix well. Spoon into greased 8-cup (2 L) casserole or bean pot. Bake in 350°F (180°C) oven for 1 hour.

Makes 6 servings.

Calories per serving: 89
Grams fat per serving: 0.6
Grams fibre per serving: 2.8

Excellent source of: Vitamins
 A and C
Good source of: Iron

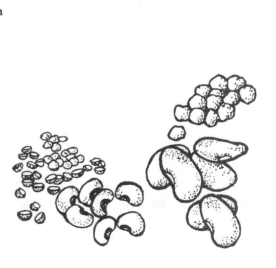

LAMB CASSOULET

Preparation time: 20 minutes
Baking time: 1-1/4 hours

Lamb sausages, introduced by New Zealand Lamb Company, are one of the lowest in fat of all sausages marketed in Canada. Teamed with lean cubes of shoulder lamb, beans and veggies, they make a great stew for cold wintry nights after a day in the fresh air.

1 lb	lamb sausages	500 g
2 tbsp	vegetable oil	25 mL
1 lb	lean shoulder lamb, cut in 1-inch (2.5 cm) cubes	500 g
1	large onion, sliced	1
1	clove garlic, minced	1
2	sweet green peppers, seeded and cut in chunks	2
4	medium carrots, thickly sliced	4
2	cans (14 oz/398 mL each) red kidney beans, undrained	2
1 cup	chicken stock	250 mL
1 tsp	dried basil	5 mL
1/2 tsp	salt	2 mL
1/4 tsp	freshly ground pepper	1 mL

If lamb sausages are unavailable for Lamb Cassoulet, use a brand of sausages that is labelled lighter in fat or calories, or reduce the amount to 1/2 lb (250 g) of regular sausages.

Dried kidney beans may be substituted for canned, see chart on page 173 for soaking times. Increase the chicken stock to 1-1/2 cups (375 mL).

☐ In large heavy skillet, brown sausages over medium heat. Cut into 1/2-inch (1 cm) thick slices; place in greased 12-cup (3 L) ovenproof casserole or Dutch oven.

☐ Add oil to skillet; brown lamb cubes along with onion and garlic, about 5 minutes. Add green peppers and carrots; cook for 1 minute longer.

☐ With slotted spoon, transfer meat and vegetables to sausages in casserole; stir in beans, chicken stock, basil, salt and pepper. Cover and bake in 350°F (180°C) oven for 1 hour and 15 minutes.

Makes 8 servings.

Calories per serving: 265
Grams fat per serving: 16.5
Grams fibre per serving: 5.1

Excellent source of: Vitamins A and C
Good source of: Phosphorus, iron and niacin

POT ROAST WITH GINGERED FRUIT AND SWEET POTATOES

Preparation time: 15 minutes
Roasting time: 1 hour and
40 minutes

*C*hoose a lean boneless pot roast, preferably short rib or chuck, for this complete dinner in one dish.

1 cup	**apple juice**	250 mL
1/2 cup	**dried figs**	125 mL
3	**thin slices gingerroot**	3
1 tbsp	**lemon juice**	15 mL
1/4 tsp	**cinnamon**	1 mL
3 lb	**boneless pot roast**	1.5 kg
1	**large onion, sliced**	1
2 or 3	**sweet potatoes, cut in chunks (1-1/4 lb/625 g)**	2 or 3
1/2 cup	**dried apricots**	125 mL

To make pot roast as lean in fat as possible, trim all visible fat from the meat. Use a heavy pan with a nonstick surface to brown meat or spray the pan with a low-calorie vegetable coating (like Pam) to prevent the meat from sticking.

☐ In bowl, mix together apple juice, figs, gingerroot, lemon juice and cinnamon; set aside.

☐ In deep flameproof casserole or Dutch oven, brown meat well on all sides over medium-high heat. Remove roast and set aside. Add onion to pan and brown lightly; drain off excess fat. Return meat to pan; add fruit mixture.

☐ Cover and roast in 300°F (150°C) oven for 1 hour. Turn meat, spooning juices over. Add sweet potato chunks and apricots; cover and roast for 20 minutes. Turn potato chunks; roast for 20 minutes longer or until meat is tender.

☐ Remove roast to warm platter; discard gingerroot. With slotted spoon, arrange fruit and potatoes around meat; keep warm. Boil liquid remaining in pan over medium-high heat until reduced to about 1-1/4 cups (300 mL). Spoon over meat and serve.

Makes 8 servings.

Calories per serving: 363
Grams fat per serving: 12.1
Grams fibre per serving: 4.1

Excellent source of: Vitamins A
and C, iron and niacin
Good source of: Phosphorus

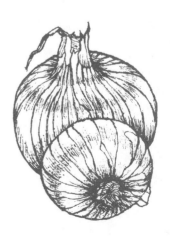

BAKED BEANS

Standing time: 1 hour or overnight
Preparation time: 1 hour
Baking time: 7 hours

Tried and true, this is the classic recipe for baked beans. You can reduce fat by using less salt pork — or none at all.

4 cups	white pea (navy) beans	1 L
1/2 cup	packed brown sugar	125 mL
1/2 cup	molasses	125 mL
1/2 cup	ketchup	125 mL
1	large apple, peeled and chopped	1
1 tsp	salt	5 mL
1 tsp	dry mustard	5 mL
4	whole cloves	4
1	large onion	1
1/2 lb	salt pork (as lean as possible)	250 g

☐ Soak beans overnight or by the quick-soak method on page 173; drain and place in large saucepan.

☐ Cover beans with fresh water; bring to boil. Reduce heat and simmer, covered, for 1 hour. Drain, reserving cooking liquid. Place beans in 12-cup (3 L) bean pot or casserole.

☐ Combine brown sugar, molasses, ketchup, apple, salt and mustard. Mix with beans, adding enough reserved cooking liquid to cover beans. Stick cloves in onion; bury in beans. Push salt pork into beans, leaving just rind exposed.

☐ Cover and bake in 250°F (120°C) oven for 6 hours, adding just enough reserved cooking liquid, if necessary, to keep beans from drying out. Uncover and bake for 1 hour longer or until beans are tender.

Makes 10 servings.

Calories per serving: 424
Grams fat per serving: 16.3
Grams fibre per serving: 12.7

Excellent source of: Iron
Good source of: Phosphorus and thiamine

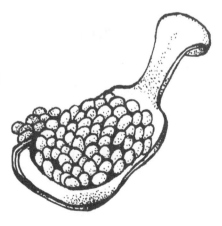

COMPANY CHILI

Preparation time: 10 minutes
Cooking time: 1-1/4 hours

*T*here are as many recipes for good chili as there are kinds of beans. This is the way we like this dish on a cold wintry night at the cottage.

1 tbsp	vegetable oil	15 mL
1	large onion, chopped	1
1	clove garlic, chopped	1
1	small sweet green pepper, chopped	1
1/2 lb	mushrooms, sliced	250 g
1 lb	lean ground beef	500 g
2	cans (14 oz/398 mL) kidney beans	2
1	can (28 oz/796 mL) tomatoes	1
1	can (7-1/2 oz/213 mL) tomato sauce	1
1 tbsp	(approx) chili powder	15 mL
1 tsp	salt	5 mL
	Cayenne pepper	

☐ In large saucepan, heat oil over medium-high heat; sauté onion and garlic for 5 minutes or until onion is softened but not browned. Add green pepper and mushrooms; cook, stirring occasionally, for 5 minutes. With slotted spoon, remove vegetables and set aside.

☐ Add beef to saucepan and cook, breaking up with wooden spoon, just until browned and no pink remains; drain off any excess fat. Add undrained kidney beans and tomatoes, tomato sauce, chili powder, salt and reserved vegetables. Bring to boil; reduce heat and simmer, covered, for about 1 hour or until flavors have mellowed and mixture has thickened. Season with more chili pepper or cayenne pepper to taste.

Makes 8 servings.

Calories per serving: 207
Grams fat per serving: 6.5
Grams fibre per serving: 7.1

Excellent source of: Iron,
vitamin C and niacin
Good source of: Phosphorus
and vitamin A

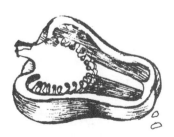

CONFETTI MEAT LOAF

Preparation time: 10 minutes
Baking time: 1 hour and
20 minutes

*O*ne of life's most comforting foods, meat loaf makes a wonderful supper when teamed with green beans or Brussels sprouts. If you're lucky enough to have any leftovers, serve this easy-to-slice meat loaf cold with a spinach and mushroom salad, or as a delicious filling for sandwiches.

1 lb	lean ground beef	500 g
1/2 lb	ground pork	250 g
1	medium onion, chopped	1
1	egg	1
1-1/2 cups	grated carrots	375 mL
1 cup	100% Bran cereal	250 mL
1/2 cup	ketchup	125 mL
1/4 cup	chopped fresh parsley	50 mL
1 tsp	salt	5 mL
1/2 tsp	dried thyme	2 mL
	Freshly ground pepper	
1 tbsp	packed brown sugar	15 mL
Dash	hot pepper sauce	Dash

Make this light French dressing for a spinach and mushroom salad: In a jar with a tight-fitting lid, combine 1/2 cup (125 mL) tomato juice, 2 tbsp (25 mL) each vinegar and vegetable oil, 1 tsp (5 mL) each salt, minced onion and Worcestershire sauce, 1/2 tsp (2 mL) dry mustard and a dash of hot pepper sauce. Store in the refrigerator. Shake well before using. Makes 3/4 cup (175 mL). Each 1 tbsp (15 mL) contains 21 calories and only 2.2 grams of fat.

☐ In large bowl, combine beef, pork, onion, egg, carrots, bran cereal, 1/4 cup (50 mL) of the ketchup, parsley, salt, thyme, and pepper to taste; mix thoroughly. Press into greased 9- x 5-inch (2 L) loaf pan.

☐ Bake in 350°F (180°C) oven for 1 hour. Drain any excess fat from pan. Mix together remaining ketchup, brown sugar and hot pepper sauce; spoon over top of meat loaf. Return to oven and bake for 30 minutes longer.

Makes 6 servings.

Calories per serving: 295
Grams fat per serving: 12.7
Grams fibre per serving: 4.1

Excellent source of:
  Phosphorus, iron, vitamin
  A, thiamine and niacin

Notes

over: *Warm Chicken Salad with Melon (page 100).*

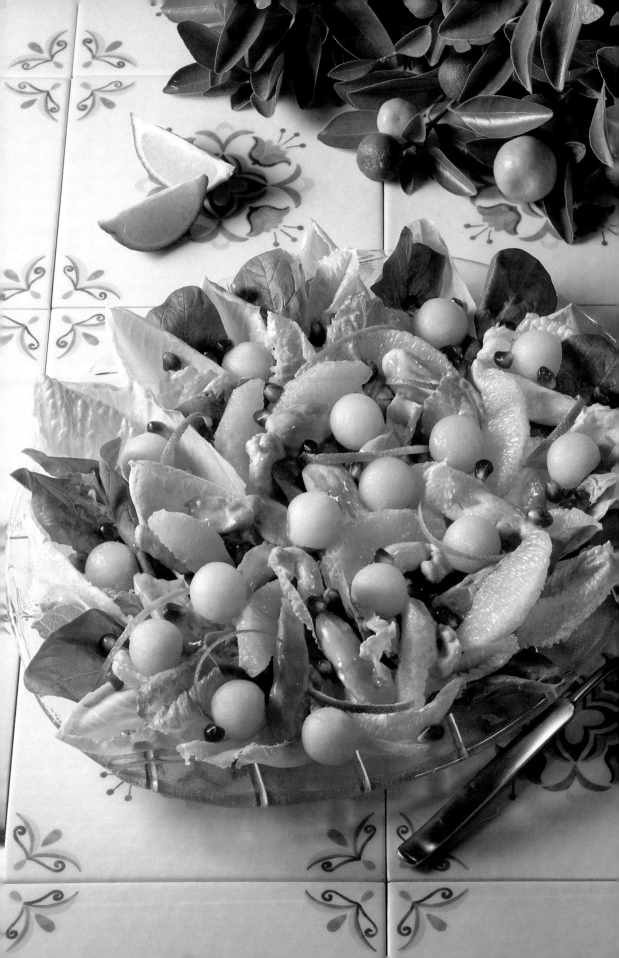

CRUNCHY CHICKEN

*I*f you want these drumsticks to be as low in fat as possible, remove the skin and all visible fat before coating. Be sure the pan is well greased or coating may stick to pan.

8	chicken drumsticks (1-1/2 lb/750 g)	8
1/2 cup	plain yogurt	125 mL
2 tsp	Dijon mustard	10 mL
2 tsp	(approx) milk	10 mL
1/2 cup	bran flake crumbs	125 mL
1/2 cup	finely chopped unsalted peanuts	125 mL
1 tsp	dried rosemary	5 mL
1/4 tsp	freshly ground pepper	1 mL
	All-purpose flour	

To make bran flake crumbs for Crunchy Chicken: In blender or food processor, crush 1 cup (250 mL) bran flake cereal until in coarse crumbs. This makes 1/2 cup (125 mL) crumbs.

☐ Rinse chicken and pat dry. In shallow dish, stir together yogurt and mustard; add up to 2 tsp (10 mL) milk if too thick to dip chicken. In separate shallow dish, combine bran flake crumbs, peanuts, rosemary and pepper.

☐ Lightly coat chicken with flour. Dip into yogurt mixture, then into crumb mixture, coating well. Place coated drumsticks on well-greased foil-lined baking sheet.

☐ Bake in 350°F (180°C) oven for 25 minutes. Turn pieces and bake for 25 minutes longer or until chicken is tender.

Makes 4 servings.

Calories per serving: 347
Grams fat per serving: 15.2
Grams fibre per serving: 2.8

Excellent source of:
 Phosphorus, thiamine
 and niacin
Good source of: Iron

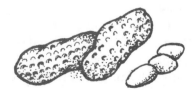

VEGETABLE CHEESE PIE

Preparation time: 35 minutes
Baking time: 45 minutes

Similar to a deep quiche but with a crunchy topping, this pie makes a perfect brunch or supper dish. Serve with crudités and bread sticks.

Crust:

3/4 cup	shredded mozzarella cheese	175 mL
1 cup	whole wheat flour	250 mL
1 cup	rolled oats	250 mL
1/4 cup	freshly grated Parmesan cheese	50 mL
1/3 cup	butter	75 mL

Filling:

2 tbsp	butter	25 mL
4 cups	shredded cabbage	1 L
1	onion, chopped	1
1	small sweet red pepper, diced	1

Custard:

3	eggs	3
1 cup	plain yogurt	250 mL
1/2 cup	shredded mozzarella cheese	125 mL
2 tbsp	freshly grated Parmesan cheese	25 mL
1/2 tsp	dried basil	2 mL
1/2 tsp	dried oregano	2 mL

Crust:

☐ In bowl, mix together mozzarella, flour, rolled oats and Parmesan. With pastry blender or your fingers, cut in butter until crumbly. Remove 1 cup (250 mL) and set aside.

☐ Press remaining crumbs over bottom and partway up side of greased 9-inch (2.5 L) springform pan. Set aside.

Filling:

☐ In skillet, melt butter; sauté cabbage, onion and red pepper just until limp, about 5 minutes. Spoon into prepared crust.

Custard:

☐ In bowl, beat eggs; blend in yogurt, mozzarella and Parmesan cheeses, basil and oregano. Pour over filling and sprinkle with reserved crumbs. Bake in 375°F (190°C) oven until puffy and set in centre, about 45 minutes. Let stand

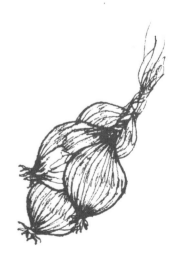

for 20 minutes. Remove side of pan and cut into 8 wedges.
Serve warm or cool.

Makes 8 servings.

Calories per serving: 304
Grams fat per serving: 17.9
Grams fibre per serving: 3.4

Excellent source of: Phosphorus
and vitamin C
Good source of: Calcium and
vitamin A

SAUCY GINGER-BAKED FISH

Preparation time: 35 minutes
Cooking time: 8 to 10 minutes

Salmon, halibut, pickerel, monkfish or any other mild-flavored firm fish is delicious flavored this way. Since sweet peppers are red, green, yellow or purple, you can mix and match the pepper strips to give a rainbow of color.

1/2 cup	**tomato sauce**	125 mL
1/4 cup	**chicken stock**	50 mL
1 tbsp	**grated fresh gingerroot**	15 mL
1 tbsp	**soy sauce**	15 mL
2 tsp	**rice vinegar**	10 mL
1 tsp	**liquid honey**	5 mL
Dash	**hot pepper sauce**	Dash
1 lb	**fish fillets or steaks**	500 g
	Salt and freshly ground pepper	
6 cups	**torn fresh spinach**	1.5 mL
1-1/2 cups	**strips of sweet red, green and yellow peppers**	375 mL
3	**green onions, sliced**	3
1 tbsp	**vegetable oil**	15 mL

☐ In low flat dish, combine tomato sauce, stock, gingerroot, soy sauce, vinegar, honey and hot pepper sauce. Add fish, turning to coat both sides. Cover with plastic wrap; marinate for 30 minutes.

☐ Place fish in well-greased baking dish; spoon sauce
generously over. Bake in 450°F (230°C) oven for 5 minutes.
Turn fish and spoon more sauce over; bake for 3 minutes
longer, depending on thickness of fish. (Fish is done when it
flakes easily when tested with fork.) Season with salt and
pepper to taste.

☐ While fish is baking, steam spinach.

☐ Meanwhile, stir-fry sweet peppers and green onions in
oil over medium-high heat just until soft but crunchy, 3 to 4
minutes. Serve fish on bed of drained spinach; spoon pepper
mixture over top.

Makes 4 servings.

Calories per serving: 234
Grams fat per serving: 10.4
Grams fibre per serving: 5.1

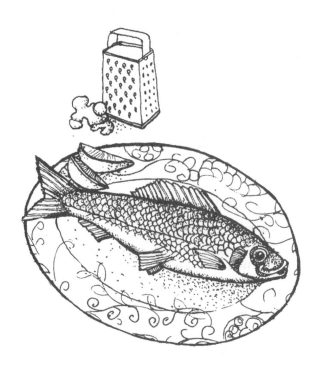

MUSTARD PORK WITH PRUNES

Preparation time: 15 minutes
Roasting time: 45 minutes

Mustard seeds are usually associated only with pickling but here they give a crunchy coating to this meat without a strong mustard flavor.

1 cup	**pitted prunes**	250 mL
1/2 cup	**chopped sweet red pepper**	125 mL
1/3 cup	**chopped green onions**	75 mL
1/4 cup	**chopped fresh parsley**	50 mL
2	**pork tenderloins (about 3/4 lb/375 g each)**	2
	Dijon mustard	
1 tsp	**coarse cracked black pepper**	5 mL
1/4 cup	**mustard seeds**	50 mL

☐ In saucepan, bring prunes and 1/2 cup (125 mL) water to boil; reduce heat and simmer for 5 minutes. Drain any excess liquid. Add red pepper, green onions and parsley; stir to mix.

☐ Make a cut in centre of side of each tenderloin; open and spread flat. Spread one piece with prune mixture. Top with second tenderloin, positioning it with thickest end on top of thinnest part of first. Tie together in 3 or 4 places. Spread thin layer of mustard over top of tenderloin.

☐ Spread mustard seeds on waxed paper; sprinkle pepper over top. Place stuffed loin, mustard-coated side down, on mustard seed mixture. Spread mustard on top (uncoated) side. Turn roll over to coat second side with seed mixture. Place in greased baking pan.

☐ Roast in 425°F (220°C) oven for 30 minutes; turn and roast for 15 minutes longer or until meat thermometer inserted in meat (not stuffing) registers 175°F (180°C).

Makes 6 servings.

Calories per serving: 242
Grams fat per serving: 6.4
Grams fibre per serving: 4.4

Excellent source of:
  Phosphorus, thiamine
  and niacin
Good source of: Iron, vitamin
  C and riboflavin

DOUBLE CORN PANCAKES

Preparation time: 10 minutes
Cooking time: 10 to 15 minutes

*T*op these light pancakes with maple syrup, but remember that the calorie count for this dish increases according to the amount of syrup used. Each tablespoon (15 mL) of maple syrup adds 50 calories.

3/4 cup	**cornmeal**	175 mL
1/2 cup	**whole wheat flour**	125 mL
1/2 tsp	**baking powder**	2 mL
1/2 tsp	**baking soda**	2 mL
1/2 tsp	**salt**	2 mL
1 cup	**(approx) buttermilk**	250 mL
1	**egg, beaten**	1
2 tbsp	**butter, melted**	25 mL
1 cup	**corn kernels, fresh or frozen and thawed**	250 mL

☐ In mixing bowl, stir together cornmeal, flour, baking powder, baking soda and salt. Stir in 1 cup (250 mL) buttermilk, egg and butter, mixing just until blended. (Batter may be lumpy.) Fold in corn.

☐ Heat lightly greased skillet or griddle over medium-high heat; pour in batter, about 1/4 cup (50 mL) for each pancake, and cook for 4 to 5 minutes or until top appears slightly dry and bubbles start to break surface. Turn pancakes and cook until second side is browned. If batter thickens on standing, thin with more buttermilk.

Makes 8 pancakes, 4 servings.

Calories per serving: 266
Grams fat per serving: 8.3
Grams fibre per serving: 3.5

Good source of: Phosphorus

BAKED POTATO PRIMAVERA

Preparation time: 10 minutes
Baking time: 45 minutes

*C*an you top this? The lowly potato is a great source of fibre and becomes a serving container for colorful fresh vegetables. Mix and match them according to the season.

4	large baking potatoes	4
1/2 cup	broccoli florets	125 mL
1/2 cup	sliced unpeeled zucchini, green or yellow	125 mL
1/2 cup	diagonally sliced carrots	125 mL
1/2 cup	snow peas	125 mL
4 tsp	butter	20 mL
1/4 cup	shredded Cheddar cheese	50 mL

Vegetables for Baked Potato Primavera should be cooked until tender-crisp, preferably steamed over as little water as possible.

For maximum fibre benefit, leave skins on vegetables when possible.

☐ Thoroughly wash and dry potatoes; pierce with fork to let steam escape during baking. Bake in 400°F (200°C) oven for 45 minutes to 1 hour or until tender.

☐ Slice off top third of each potato; scoop out some of the pulp to form pocket. (Keep unused cooked potato to stir-fry or put into a salad the next day.) Return potatoes to oven to keep warm; turn oven off.

☐ Steam broccoli, zucchini, carrots and snow peas until tender-crisp, about 2 minutes. Spoon vegetables attractively into potato pockets. Dot each with 1 tsp (5 mL) butter; sprinkle each with 1 tbsp (15 mL) cheese. Serve at once.

Makes 4 servings.

Calories per serving: 207
Grams fat per serving: 6.2
Grams fibre per serving: 3.1

Excellent source of: Vitamins A and C
Good source of: Phosphorus

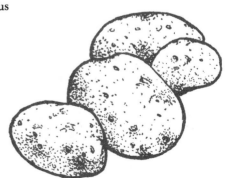

POTATO NESTS WITH PEAS AND OLIVES

Preparation time: 15 minutes
Baking time: 30 to 35 minutes

*I*f you only want to serve half of the nests, cool the remainder thoroughly after baking. Wrap them tightly and freeze the nests for up to three weeks. To reheat, bake upside down on baking sheet in 375°F (190°C) oven for 8 to 10 minutes or until hot and crisp. You can use them to hold other plain or creamed vegetables.

2 cups	**mashed potatoes (about 4 medium potatoes)**	500 mL
1/4 cup	**finely chopped onion**	50 mL
1/4 cup	**shredded mild cheese, such as Muenster, Swiss or mozzarella**	50 mL
1	**egg yolk**	1
2 tbsp	**chopped fresh parsley**	25 mL
1/4 tsp	**salt**	1 mL
1/4 tsp	**freshly ground pepper**	1 mL
3 cups	**fresh or frozen peas**	750 mL
2 tbsp	**slivered pitted black olives**	25 mL

Instead of peas, fill potato nests with a succotash mixture of 1-1/2 cups (375 mL) cooked corn, 1-1/2 cups (375 mL) cooked lima beans, 1 tbsp (15 mL) butter, and salt and pepper to taste.

☐ In bowl, mix together potatoes, onion, cheese, egg yolk, parsley, salt and pepper; divide among 12 medium or 6 large greased muffin cups, patting evenly over bottoms and up sides. Bake in 350°F (180°C) oven for 30 to 35 minutes or until golden. Let cool slightly in pans; run knife around edges and remove carefully.

☐ Meanwhile, cook peas in small amount of lightly salted boiling water; drain and toss with olives. Spoon into warm nests.

Makes 12 medium or 6 large nests, enough for 6 servings.

Calories per serving: 131
Grams fat per serving: 2.7
Grams fibre per serving: 8.6

Good source of: Vitamin C and thiamine

RATATOUILLE

Preparation time: 10 minutes
Cooking time: 15 minutes

*A*sparagus makes this an unusual vegetable side dish. If fresh asparagus is unavailable, substitute fresh green beans or peas.

2 tbsp	**vegetable oil**	25 mL
2 cups	**sliced mushrooms**	500 mL
1	**medium onion, sliced**	1
1	**clove garlic, chopped**	1
1	**sweet green pepper, sliced**	1
1	**small eggplant (about 1/2 lb/ 250 g), unpeeled and cut in 1/2-inch (1 cm) dice**	1
1/2 lb	**fresh asparagus, cut in 1-inch (2.5 cm) lengths**	250 g
1 tbsp	**chopped fresh parsley**	15 mL
1 tbsp	**chopped fresh basil or 1 tsp (5 mL) dried**	15 mL
1 tsp	**salt**	5 mL
1/4 tsp	**freshly ground pepper**	1 mL
2 cups	**cherry tomatoes, halved**	500 mL

In summertime, Ratatouille makes a delicious cold side dish. Chill in refrigerator, then drain off any excess liquid.

☐ In large skillet or wok, heat 1 tbsp (15 mL) of the oil over medium-high heat; stir-fry mushrooms, onion, garlic and green pepper for 3 to 4 minutes or until softened. With slotted spoon, remove vegetables to bowl and set aside.

☐ Heat remaining oil in skillet. Add eggplant and asparagus; stir-fry just until tender, 3 to 4 minutes. Return mushroom mixture to pan; sprinkle with parsley, basil, salt and pepper and stir well. Add tomatoes; cover and simmer for 3 minutes. Serve immediately.

Makes 6 servings.

Calories per serving: 79
Grams fat per serving: 4.8
Grams fibre per serving: 2.4

Excellent source of: Vitamin C
Good source of: Vitamin A

RUTABAGA PEAR BAKE

Preparation time: 30 minutes
Baking time: 20 minutes

*F*or years we called these big yellow globes "turnips". Now, because the small white turnips are common, this wonderful storage vegetable (hence a winter root that has become a staple) is correctly called rutabaga.

1	large rutabaga	1
1	small onion, chopped	1
2 cups	chicken stock	500 mL
1/4 cup	butter	50 mL
1/4 cup	all-purpose flour	50 mL
1-1/2 cups	milk	375 mL
1/2 tsp	salt	2 mL
Pinch	freshly grated nutmeg	Pinch
2 cups	sliced peeled pears	500 mL
1/2 cup	dry bread crumbs, preferably whole wheat	125 mL
1 tbsp	snipped fresh chives	15 mL
1 tbsp	chopped fresh parsley	15 mL
1 tbsp	butter, melted	15 mL

For a change of flavor in Rutabaga Pear Bake, use 2 cups (500 mL) peeled, sliced apples instead of the pears.

☐ Peel rutabaga; cut into quarters. Cut quarters into 1/4-inch (5 mm) thick slices. In saucepan, simmer rutabaga and onion in chicken stock for about 15 minutes or until rutabaga is tender-crisp. With slotted spoon, transfer rutabaga to greased 8-cup (2 L) shallow gratin or baking dish; set aside.

☐ Bring stock to boil and cook until reduced to 1 cup (250 mL).

☐ In another saucepan, melt 1/4 cup (50 mL) butter; blend in flour. Gradually add reduced stock along with milk, stirring constantly. Cook, stirring, until sauce thickens and comes to boil. Remove from heat; add salt and nutmeg. Taste and adjust seasoning.

☐ Add pears to rutabaga in gratin dish and toss to mix. Pour sauce over top.

☐ Mix together bread crumbs, chives, parsley and 1 tbsp (15 mL) melted butter; sprinkle over casserole. Bake in 375°F (190°C) oven for about 20 minutes or until rutabaga is fork-tender and topping is browned.

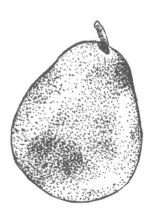

Makes 6 servings.

Calories per serving: 206
Grams fat per serving: 11.1
Grams fibre per serving: 3.5

Excellent source of: Vitamin C
Good source of: Vitamin A

STIR-FRIED SPINACH WITH LENTILS

Preparation time: 5 minutes
Cooking time: 5 minutes

*T*his combination of spinach and lentils makes a pleasant side dish to accompany beef, lamb, chicken or fish.

6 cups	fresh spinach, packed	1.5 L
1 tbsp	butter	15 mL
1 cup	cooked or canned lentils (see page 173)	250 mL
1/2 tsp	salt	2 mL
1/4 tsp	ground ginger	1 mL
	Freshly ground pepper	
1 tbsp	toasted sesame seeds	15 mL

☐ In large skillet, cook spinach over medium-high heat, in just the water clinging to leaves after washing, for 2 to 3 minutes or just until spinach barely wilts. Drain well.

☐ Add butter to skillet; stir in lentils, salt, ginger, and pepper to taste. Stir-fry until heated through. Serve at once, sprinkled with sesame seeds.

Makes 4 servings.

Calories per serving: 121
Grams fat per serving: 5.5
Grams fibre per serving: 6.7

Excellent source of: Iron and vitamin A
Good source of: Vitamin C

CURRIED WILD RICE AND PEACHES

Preparation time: 15 minutes
Cooking time: 10 minutes

Delicious with cooked shrimp, this side dish also goes well with roast pork or broiled fish or chicken. You can change the flavor by substituting apples or pears for the peaches.

1	can (14 oz/398 mL) peaches **OR** 1 cup (250 mL) chopped peeled fresh peaches and 3/4 cup (175 mL) chicken stock	1
2 tbsp	butter	25 mL
1 cup	sliced celery	250 mL
1/2 cup	chopped onion	125 mL
1 cup	cooked wild rice	250 mL
2 tsp	Dijon mustard	10 mL
1/2 tsp	curry powder	2 mL
1/2 tsp	salt	2 mL

☐ Drain and chop peaches, reserving juice; set aside.

☐ In skillet, melt butter over medium-high heat; sauté celery and onion until softened, 3 to 4 minutes. Add cooked rice, reserved peach juice (or chicken stock if using fresh peaches), mustard, curry powder and salt. Cover and simmer for 10 minutes.

☐ Add chopped peaches and heat through.

Makes 4 servings.

Calories per serving: 250
Grams fat per serving: 6.1
Grams fibre per serving: 2.1

Good source of: Niacin, phosphorus and iron

To cook wild rice: Rinse rice well under cold running water. In saucepan, cover rice with three times as much boiling water as rice. Simmer gently, covered, for about 45 minutes or until rice is tender but chewy. Drain. (Wild rice triples in volume when cooked.)

Quick-boil method: Rinse rice well under cold running water. In saucepan, cover rice with three times as much boiling water as rice. Boil for 5 minutes; remove from heat and let stand for 1 hour. (This is a great way to precook rice in the morning to use in a rush-hour supper dish.)

MUSHROOM BARLEY BAKE

Preparation time: 40 minutes
Baking time: 20 to 25
minutes

*F*or a festive touch, add 1 tbsp (15 mL) chopped pimiento to this intriguing side dish and sprinkle with 1/4 cup (50 mL) toasted slivered almonds.

1 cup	**barley**	250 mL
2 tbsp	**butter**	25 mL
3-1/2 cups	**(approx) chicken stock**	875 mL
2	**green onions, chopped**	2
1	**clove garlic, minced (optional)**	1
1 cup	**sliced mushrooms**	250 mL
1 tbsp	**chopped fresh parsley**	15 mL
1 tsp	**granulated sugar**	5 mL
	Salt and freshly ground pepper	

☐ Wash barley in cold water; drain well. In heavy saucepan, melt 1 tbsp (15 mL) of the butter over medium heat; add barley and cook, stirring, until barley begins to brown, about 5 minutes.

☐ Add chicken stock and bring to boil. Cover and reduce heat until boiling gently; cook until barley is crunchy and tender and liquid has been absorbed, about 35 minutes. (Add more stock or water during cooking, if necessary.)

☐ In skillet, melt remaining butter over medium heat; sauté onions, garlic, if using, and mushrooms for 2 minutes. Stir into barley along with parsley, sugar, and salt and pepper to taste. Spoon into greased 6-cup (1.5 L) casserole. (Recipe can be prepared to this point, covered and refrigerated for up to 8 hours.)

☐ Bake in 350°F (180°C) oven for 20 to 25 minutes (or longer if directly from refrigerator) or until heated through.

Makes 6 servings.

Calories per serving: 174   Good source of: Niacin
Grams fat per serving: 4.8
Grams fibre per serving: 2.5

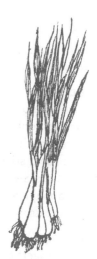

BAKED MUSTARD CABBAGE

Preparation time: 20 minutes
Baking time: 20 minutes

*D*elicious with roast chicken, bake this dish along with the chicken for a complete oven meal.

8 cups	**coarsely chopped cabbage (about 1-1/2 lb/750 g)**	2 L
Sauce:		
2 tbsp	**butter**	25 mL
3 tbsp	**all-purpose flour**	50 mL
2 cups	**milk**	500 mL
2 tbsp	**Dijon mustard**	25 mL
1 tsp	**Worcestershire sauce**	5 mL
1/2 tsp	**salt**	2 mL
1/4 tsp	**white pepper**	1 mL
1/4 tsp	**freshly grated nutmeg**	1 mL
Dash	**hot pepper sauce**	Dash
1 cup	**shredded Swiss cheese (about 3 oz/90 g)**	250 mL
Topping:		
1 cup	**dry bread crumbs**	250 mL
2 tbsp	**freshly grated Parmesan cheese**	25 mL
1 tbsp	**butter, melted**	25 mL

☐ In large pot of lightly salted boiling water, blanch cabbage. (It should be limp but bright green and slightly crisp.) Drain and refresh under cold running water. Drain well.

Sauce:
☐ In saucepan, melt butter over medium heat; blend in flour and cook until bubbly. Stir in milk, mustard, Worcestershire sauce, salt, pepper, nutmeg and hot pepper sauce; cook, stirring, until mixture thickens and comes to boil. Stir in Swiss cheese and heat just until melted. Pour over cabbage and toss. Spoon into greased 8-cup (2 L) shallow casserole dish.

Topping:
☐ Mix together bread crumbs, Parmesan cheese and butter; sprinkle over cabbage mixture. Bake in 350°F

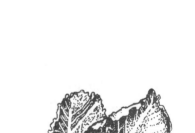

(180°C) oven for about 20 minutes or until brown and bubbly.

Makes 6 servings.

Calories per serving: 255
Grams fat per serving: 12.8
Grams fibre per serving: 3.9

Excellent source of: Calcium
   and vitamin C
Good source of: Phosphorus

BARLEY PILAF

Preparation time: 10 minutes
Cooking time: 45 minutes

A pleasant change from potatoes or rice, this pilaf goes well with meat, chicken or fish.

1 cup	barley	250 mL
2 tbsp	butter	25 mL
1	small onion, chopped	1
1	stalk celery, chopped	1
3 cups	boiling water	750 mL
1 tsp	salt	5 mL
1 tsp	dried thyme	5 mL

☐ Spread barley on baking sheet; broil for 2 to 3 minutes or until toasted and lightly browned, stirring occasionally. (Alternatively, bake in 375°F/190°C oven for 6 to 8 minutes, stirring occasionally.)

☐ In large saucepan, melt butter; sauté onion and celery for 2 minutes or until softened and fragrant. Stir in toasted barley. Add boiling water, salt and thyme; cover and simmer for 45 minutes or until barley is tender.

Makes 6 servings.

Calories per serving: 147
Grams fat per serving: 4
Grams fibre per serving: 2.3

Notes

Notes

over: *Pasta Niçoise (page 103).*

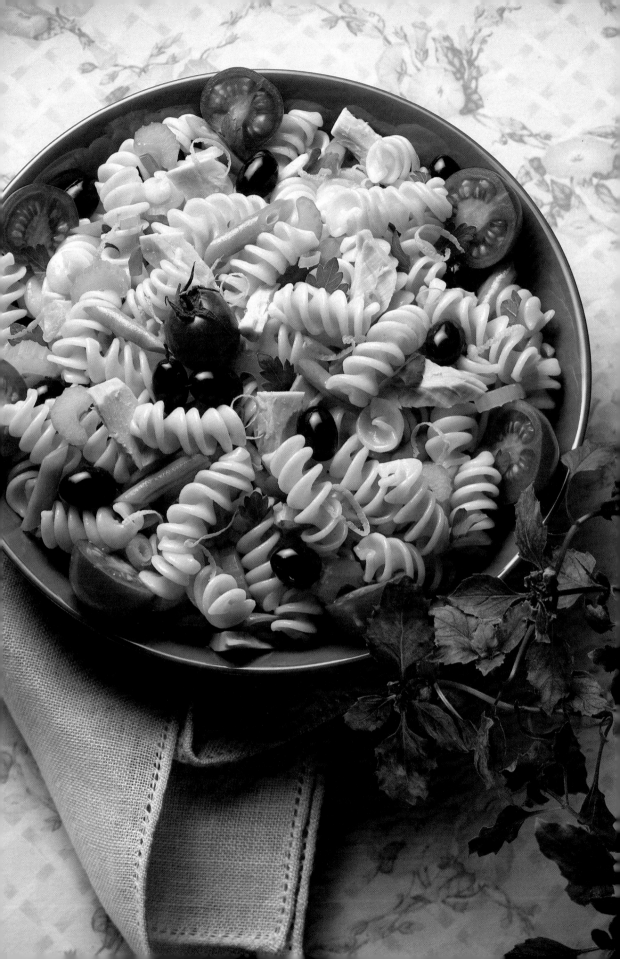

Breads and Baking

Whole-grain flour—wheat, rye, graham or corn—is one of the best ways to incorporate fibre into your diet. Try to use whole wheat flour as part of the flour in all your yeast breads, quick breads, cookies and cakes. All-purpose or white flour loses nutrients and fibre during refining and while most nutrients are added back into the final product, the fibre is not replaced. Nutrition experts have been urging us to eat whole-grain cereals and flour for years, knowing that the fibre in them is important.

Besides adding a whole-grain flour, you can increase fibre in your baked goods by adding dried fruit, nuts, seeds, natural bran and whole-grain cereals.

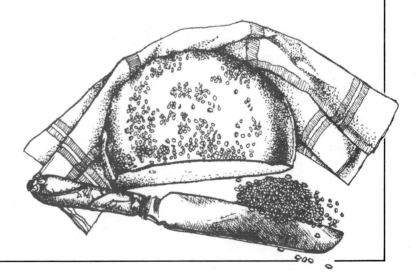

PEPPERY CORN BREAD

Preparation time: 10 minutes
Baking time: 30 to 35
minutes

*T*his savory corn bread has an interesting bite. Use less jalapeño peppers, if desired, or omit completely. Serve cut into squares.

1 cup	**cornmeal**	250 mL
1/2 cup	**whole wheat flour**	125 mL
1/2 cup	**all-purpose flour**	125 mL
1 tbsp	**baking powder**	15 mL
1/2 tsp	**baking soda**	2 mL
1/2 tsp	**salt**	2 mL
3	**eggs**	3
1 cup	**plain yogurt**	250 mL
1/3 cup	**butter, melted**	75 mL
1	**can (10 oz/284 mL) cream-style corn**	1
1 tbsp	**finely chopped jalapeño peppers**	15 mL
1 cup	**shredded Cheddar cheese (about 4 oz/125 g)**	250 mL

Handle hot peppers with care. The volatile oil released from the seeds can be very irritating. Be careful not to handle peppers and then rub your eyes.

☐ In large bowl, combine cornmeal, whole wheat and all-purpose flours, baking powder, baking soda and salt.

☐ In separate bowl, beat eggs until light and frothy. Beat in yogurt, butter and corn. Add to dry ingredients and mix well. Stir in jalapeño peppers and cheese.

☐ Pour batter into greased 9-inch (2.5 L) square cake pan. Bake in 375°F (190°C) oven for 35 to 40 minutes or until tester inserted in centre comes out clean. Let cool slightly in pan. Cut into 16 squares and serve warm.

Makes 16 squares.

Calories per square: 157
Grams fat per square: 7.6
Grams fibre per square: 2

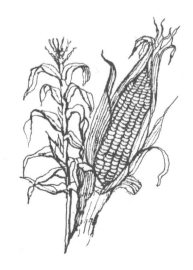

OATMEAL RAISIN SCONES

*W*e usually think of whole wheat when we think of whole grain, but rolled oats (oatmeal) is a whole grain cereal as well. Serve these melt-in-your-mouth scones warm with marmalade or jam.

3/4 cup	**all-purpose flour**	175 mL
3/4 cup	**whole wheat flour**	175 mL
1 cup	**quick-cooking rolled oats**	250 mL
1 tsp	**baking soda**	5 mL
1/2 tsp	**salt**	2 mL
1/4 cup	**butter, softened**	50 mL
1/3 cup	**raisins or currants**	75 mL
3/4 cup	**buttermilk or soured milk**	175 mL

To sour milk for Oatmeal Raisin Scones: Place 2 tsp (10 mL) lemon juice or vinegar in a measuring cup. Add milk to the 3/4 cup (175 mL) level. Let stand for 10 minutes, then stir.

☐ In large bowl, combine all-purpose and whole wheat flours, rolled oats, baking soda and salt. With pastry blender or 2 knives, cut in butter until mixture resembles cornmeal. Stir in raisins. With fork, stir in buttermilk just until moistened. Divide dough in half.

☐ With lightly floured hands, pat out each portion onto greased baking sheet, forming circle about 1/2 inch (1 cm) thick. Lightly score each circle into quarters but do not cut through.

☐ Bake in 400°F (200°C) oven for about 15 minutes or until golden brown.

Makes 8 scones.

Calories per scone: 196
Grams fat per scone: 6.7
Grams fibre per scone: 2.5

PUMPERNICKEL CARAWAY BREAD

Preparation time: 20 minutes
Rising time: 3 hours
Baking time: 40 minutes

*F*or a shiny crust, brush loaf with lightly beaten egg white just before baking. For a soft crust, brush loaf with oil or melted butter as soon as it comes out of the oven.

1 tsp	**granulated sugar**	5 mL
1-1/2 cups	**lukewarm water**	375 mL
1	**package active dry yeast or 1 tbsp (15 mL)**	1
2 cups	**rye flour**	500 mL
1/3 cup	**molasses**	75 mL
2 tbsp	**vegetable oil**	25 mL
2 tsp	**salt**	10 mL
2 tsp	**caraway seeds**	10 mL
2 cups	**whole wheat flour**	500 mL
2 cups	**(approx) all-purpose flour**	500 mL
	Cornmeal for baking sheet	

☐ In large bowl, dissolve sugar in lukewarm water. Sprinkle yeast over top and let stand for 10 minutes or until frothy. Stir well.

☐ Add rye flour, molasses, oil, salt and caraway seeds; stir well. Gradually add whole wheat flour and 1 cup (250 mL) of the all-purpose flour, stirring vigorously to mix well. Turn out onto floured surface and knead for about 8 minutes, working in enough of the remaining all-purpose flour to make smooth stiff dough.

☐ Place dough in large greased bowl, turning to grease all over. Cover with greased plastic wrap and let rise until doubled in bulk, about 2 hours.

☐ Punch dough down and shape into 2 rounds or oblongs. Place on greased baking sheets lightly dusted with cornmeal. Cover with greased plastic wrap and let rise for 1 hour or until nearly doubled in bulk. Bake in 425°F (220°C) oven for 10 minutes. Reduce heat to 350°F (180°C) and bake for 30 minutes longer or until loaves sound hollow when tapped on bottom.

Makes 2 loaves, 16 slices each, 2 slices per serving.

Calories per serving: 173
Grams fat per serving: 2.3
Grams fibre per serving: 2.5

Good source of: Iron

WHOLE WHEAT BISCUITS

*P*erfect accompaniments for a hearty soup or salad supper, these biscuits are tasty substitutes for the dumplings in the Steak and Kidney Stew on page 112.

1 cup	**whole wheat flour**	250 mL
1 cup	**all-purpose flour**	250 mL
1 tbsp	**baking powder**	15 mL
1 tsp	**baking soda**	5 mL
1/4 tsp	**salt**	1 mL
1/4 cup	**shortening**	50 mL
3/4 cup	**buttermilk**	175 mL

For pull-apart, soft biscuits, bake them with sides touching. For crisp-sided biscuits, bake them at least 1 inch (2.5 cm) apart on baking sheet.

☐ In bowl, mix together whole wheat and all-purpose flours, baking powder, baking soda and salt. With pastry blender or 2 knives, cut in shortening until mixture resembles crumbs. Gradually add buttermilk, stirring with fork to make soft but not sticky dough.

☐ Turn out onto lightly floured surface. Knead lightly 10 or 12 times; pat or roll out to 3/4-inch (2 cm) thickness. With floured 2-inch (5 cm) cutter, cut out rounds and place on lightly greased baking sheet. Bake in 425°F (220°C) oven for 15 to 20 minutes or until lightly browned.

Makes 10 biscuits.

Calories per biscuit: 136
Grams fat per biscuit: 5.5
Grams fibre per biscuit: 1.5

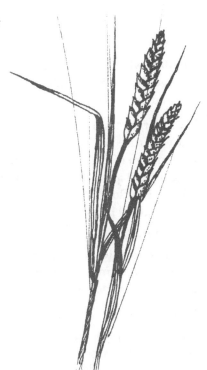

ONION CASSEROLE BREAD

Preparation time: 15 minutes
Rising time: 1-3/4 hours
Baking time: 50 minutes

*T*he wonderful aroma of this bread baking will bring everyone to the kitchen in anticipation. Serve warm in wedges with a big pot of Baked Beans (page 118) or Lima Bean Bake (page 115) and a crisp green salad.

1 tsp	granulated sugar	5 mL
1/4 cup	lukewarm water	50 mL
1	package active dry yeast or 1 tbsp (15 mL)	1
1 cup	cottage cheese	250 mL
2 tbsp	granulated sugar	25 mL
1 tbsp	butter	15 mL
2 tsp	fennel seed, dill seed or aniseed	10 mL
1 tsp	salt	5 mL
1	small onion, finely chopped	1
1	egg, beaten	1
1-1/2 cups	whole wheat flour	375 mL
1 cup	(approx) all-purpose flour	250 mL

To use whole wheat flour in bread recipes calling for all-purpose flour, substitute up to two-thirds the amount of flour. Whole wheat flour has less protein and gluten and tends to make a bread with a more compact texture. Rising times may be longer when using whole wheat flour.

☐ Dissolve 1 tsp (5 mL) sugar in lukewarm water. Sprinkle yeast over top and let stand for 10 minutes or until frothy. Stir well.

☐ Meanwhile, in saucepan over low heat, stir together cottage cheese, 2 tbsp (25 mL) sugar, butter, fennel seed, salt and onion; heat just until lukewarm.

☐ In large mixing bowl, combine cheese mixture with yeast mixture and egg. Gradually add whole wheat flour and enough of the all-purpose flour to make stiff dough, beating well after each addition. (You may not need all the all-purpose flour.) Cover dough with tea towel and let rise until doubled in bulk, about 1 hour.

☐ Punch dough down and turn into well-greased 6-cup (1.5 L) casserole. Let rise until doubled in bulk, about 45 minutes. Bake in 350°F (180°C) oven for 50 minutes or until well browned. Cut into 12 wedges to serve.

Makes 1 loaf, 12 wedges.

Calories per wedge: 130
Grams fat per wedge: 2.2
Grams fibre per wedge: 2.1

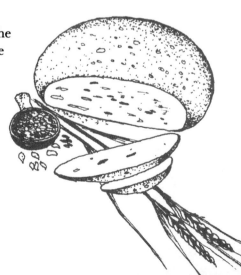

CARAWAY CRISPS

Preparation time: 20 minutes
Baking time: 8 to 10 minutes

*T*hese crispy crackerlike wafers go particularly well with soups or salads.

2 cups	**whole wheat flour**	500 mL
1/2 cup	**cornmeal**	125 mL
2 tbsp	**granulated sugar**	25 mL
1/2 tsp	**baking soda**	2 mL
1/2 tsp	**salt**	2 mL
1/4 cup	**butter**	50 mL
1/2 cup	**ice-cold water**	125 mL
2 tbsp	**vinegar**	25 mL
2 tbsp	**(approx) caraway seeds**	25 mL

☐ In large bowl, mix together flour, cornmeal, sugar, baking soda and salt. Using pastry blender or two knives, cut in butter until mixture resembles coarse crumbs. Stir in water and vinegar. With hands, knead until well mixed.

☐ Roll rounded tablespoonfuls (15 mL) of dough into small balls. On lightly floured surface, roll out each ball into very thin circle about 4 inches (10 cm) in diameter. Sprinkle each with a few caraway seeds; press seeds into dough with rolling pin.

☐ Transfer rounds to ungreased baking sheets; bake in 375°F (190°C) oven for 8 to 10 minutes or until light golden. Transfer to wire racks to let cool. Store in tightly covered container.

Makes about 32 crisps.

Calories per crisp: 48
Grams fat per crisp: 1.6
Grams fibre per crisp: 0.8

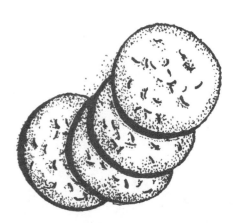

ORANGE DATE MUFFINS

Preparation time: 15 minutes
Baking time: 15 to 20 minutes

*P*aper baking cups set in muffin cups save greasing pans. They speed clean-up time as well!

1-1/4 cups	whole wheat flour	300 mL
1 cup	all-purpose flour	250 mL
3/4 cup	lightly packed brown sugar	175 mL
2 tsp	baking powder	10 mL
1 tsp	baking soda	5 mL
1/2 tsp	salt	2 mL
3/4 cup	chopped dates	175 mL
1 tsp	grated orange rind	5 mL
2	eggs	2
1/2 cup	orange juice	125 mL
1/3 cup	butter, melted	75 mL

☐ In mixing bowl, stir together whole wheat and all-purpose flours, sugar, baking powder, baking soda and salt. Stir in dates and orange rind.

☐ In separate bowl, beat eggs; blend in orange juice and melted butter. With fork, stir into dry ingredients just until moistened.

☐ Spoon batter into 12 greased or paper-lined muffin cups, filling each two-thirds full. Bake in 400°F (200°C) oven for 15 to 20 minutes or until firm to the touch.

Makes 12 large muffins.

Calories per muffin: 224
Grams fat per muffin: 6.2
Grams fibre per muffin: 2.6

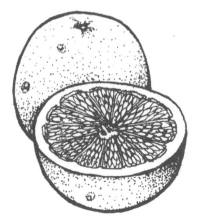

BLUEBERRY BRAN MUFFINS

*I*f fresh or frozen blueberries are unavailable, raisins are a tasty substitute.

1 cup	**natural bran**	250 mL
1/2 cup	**rolled oats**	125 mL
1/3 cup	**wheat germ**	75 mL
1/2 tsp	**cinnamon**	2 mL
1/4 tsp	**salt**	1 mL
1 cup	**buttermilk or soured milk**	250 mL
1/3 cup	**liquid honey**	75 mL
1	**egg, lightly beaten**	1
1/4 cup	**vegetable oil**	50 mL
1/2 cup	**all-purpose flour**	125 mL
1 tsp	**baking powder**	5 mL
1/2 tsp	**baking soda**	2 mL
1/2 cup	**blueberries**	125 mL
Topping:		
1/4 cup	**packed brown sugar**	50 mL
1/4 cup	**rolled oats**	50 mL
2 tbsp	**all-purpose flour**	25 mL
2 tbsp	**butter, melted**	25 mL

Bran is the outside coating of a whole grain.

Natural bran (wheat or oats) is a fine milling of 100% unprocessed bran. It is usually used in baking, much like flour.

100% Bran cereal, **All-Bran** and **Bran Buds** are cereals made of bran that has been cooked with flavorings, then ground, dried and extruded in their familiar shapes.

Bran Flakes is a cereal, a mixture of whole wheat and wheat bran. It is 40% bran.

☐ In bowl, combine bran, oats, wheat germ, cinnamon and salt; stir in buttermilk and let stand for 30 minutes.

☐ Add honey, egg and oil, mixing well. Stir together flour, baking powder and baking soda; add to bran mixture all at once, stirring just to moisten. Fold in blueberries. Spoon into 12 large greased muffin tins, filling each about two-thirds full.

Topping:
☐ Combine sugar, rolled oats, flour and butter. Sprinkle over muffins and bake in 375°F (190°C) oven for 20 to 25 minutes or until firm to the touch.

Makes 12 muffins.

Calories per muffin: 185
Grams fat per muffin: 7.6
Grams fibre per muffin: 2.9

Good source of: Phosphorus and thiamine

NO-KNEAD OATMEAL BATTER BREAD

Preparation time: 15 minutes
Rising time: 1-1/2 hours
Baking time: 40 minutes

*T*he tender texture of this small loaf makes the bread a wonderful breakfast treat when sliced and toasted under the broiler or in the toaster oven.

3/4 cup	**boiling water**	175 mL
1/2 cup	**rolled oats**	125 mL
1/4 cup	**shortening**	50 mL
1/4 cup	**liquid honey**	50 mL
1 tsp	**salt**	5 mL
1 tsp	**granulated sugar**	5 mL
1/4 cup	**lukewarm water**	50 mL
1	**package active dry yeast or 1 tbsp (15 mL)**	1
1	**egg, lightly beaten**	1
1-1/2 cups	**all-purpose flour**	375 mL
1 cup	**whole wheat flour**	250 mL
1/4 cup	**skim milk powder**	50 mL

☐ In large bowl, combine boiling water, rolled oats, shortening, honey and salt; stir until shortening has melted. Let cool to lukewarm.

☐ Dissolve sugar in lukewarm water; sprinkle yeast over and let stand for 10 minutes or until frothy. Stir well.

☐ Add beaten egg to rolled oats mixture along with half of the all-purpose flour, yeast mixture, whole wheat flour and skim milk powder. Beat vigorously with wooden spoon for 2 minutes. Add remaining all-purpose flour and mix well (you may want to use your hands). Batter will be sticky.

☐ Pat into greased 8- x 4-inch (1.5 L) loaf pan using greased hands to smooth top. Cover with greased plastic wrap and let rise until dough has doubled in bulk and has almost reached top of pan, about 1-1/2 hours.

☐ Bake in 375°F (190°C) oven for 40 minutes or until loaf is brown and sounds hollow when tapped on bottom.

Makes 16 slices, 2 slices per serving.

Calories per serving: 258   Good source of: Thiamine
Grams fat per serving: 7.8
Grams fibre per serving: 2.6

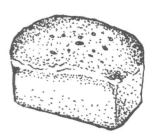

RASPBERRY TEA MUFFINS

Preparation time: 15 minutes
Baking time: 25 to 30
minutes

*F*reshly picked raspberries give a tangy flavor to these tea muffins. In winter, use individually frozen unsweetened raspberries; add them to the batter without thawing first.

1/2 cup	plain yogurt	125 mL
1/4 cup	vegetable oil	50 mL
1	egg	1
1 cup	raspberries	250 mL
2/3 cup	whole wheat flour	150 mL
2/3 cup	all-purpose flour	150 mL
2/3 cup	packed brown sugar	150 mL
1/2 tsp	baking soda	2 mL
1/4 tsp	salt	1 mL
1/2 cup	chopped nuts	125 mL
Topping:		
3 tbsp	packed brown sugar	50 mL
3 tbsp	chopped nuts	50 mL
2 tsp	butter, melted	10 mL
1/2 tsp	cinnamon	2 mL

For a change of pace, use freshly picked diced rhubarb instead of the raspberries in Raspberry Tea Muffins. In winter, use frozen rhubarb, thawed only enough to break up.

Topping:

☐ In small bowl, combine brown sugar, nuts, butter and cinnamon; set aside.

☐ In separate small bowl, blend together yogurt, oil and egg; set aside.

☐ In large bowl, stir together raspberries, whole wheat and all-purpose flours, brown sugar, baking soda and salt. With fork, stir in yogurt mixture just until moistened; fold in nuts. Spoon into 12 greased muffin cups, filling each two-thirds full.

☐ Spoon a little topping onto each muffin. Bake in 350°F (180°C) oven for 25 to 30 minutes or until firm to the touch.

Makes 12 muffins.

Calories per muffin: 192
Grams fat per muffin: 9.2
Grams fibre per muffin: 2

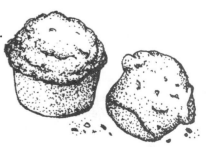

CARROT CAKE

Preparation time: 15 minutes
Baking time: 60 to 70 minutes

*F*or an attractive presentation, you can bake this cake in a 9-inch (3 L) tube or Bundt pan. Let it cool for 10 minutes before removing pan.

1 cup	whole wheat flour	250 mL
1 cup	all-purpose flour	250 mL
2 tsp	baking powder	10 mL
2 tsp	cinnamon	10 mL
1 tsp	baking soda	5 mL
1 tsp	salt	5 mL
1/2 tsp	ground cloves	2 mL
1/2 tsp	freshly grated nutmeg	2 mL
3	eggs	3
1 cup	vegetable oil	250 mL
1 cup	packed brown sugar	250 mL
1/2 cup	granulated sugar	125 mL
2-1/2 cups	grated raw carrots	625 mL
1 cup	raisins	250 mL
3/4 cup	chopped nuts	175 mL
1 tbsp	icing sugar	15 mL

☐ Mix together whole wheat and all-purpose flours, baking powder, cinnamon, baking soda, salt, cloves and nutmeg. Set aside.

☐ In large bowl, beat together eggs, oil, and brown and granulated sugars. Stir in dry ingredients. Add carrots, raisins and nuts; mix well.

☐ Pour batter into greased and floured 13- x 9-inch (3.5 L) cake pan. Bake in 350°F (180°C) oven for 55 minutes or until tester inserted in centre comes out clean. Let cool, then dust with icing sugar. Cut into 20 squares to serve.

Makes 20 squares.

Calories per square: 266
Grams fat per square: 13.8
Grams fibre per square: 2

Excellent source of: Vitamin A

CHUNKY FRUIT LOAF

Preparation time: 20 minutes
Baking time: 50 to 60 minutes

*S*tudded with fruits and nuts, this easy-to-make loaf is delicious enough to be a simplified Christmas cake, yet contains no butter or shortening.

1-1/2 cups	**pitted dates, halved**	375 mL
1-1/2 cups	**shelled Brazil nuts**	375 mL
1/2 cup	**dried apricots, halved**	125 mL
1/2 cup	**golden raisins**	125 mL
1/2 cup	**lightly packed brown sugar**	125 mL
1/2 cup	**all-purpose flour**	125 mL
1/2 tsp	**baking powder**	2 mL
Pinch	**salt**	Pinch
2	**eggs**	2
1/2 tsp	**vanilla**	2 mL

As a Christmas cake, Chunky Fruit Loaf mellows if wrapped in brandy- or sherry-soaked cheesecloth. Overwrap with plastic wrap or foil and store in the refrigerator.

☐ In large bowl, mix together dates, nuts, apricots and raisins. Stir together sugar, flour, baking powder and salt. Add to fruit mixture; stir to mix well.

☐ Beat eggs with vanilla; add to fruit mixture, stirring until completely blended. Spoon batter into well-greased and floured 8- x 4-inch (1.5 L) loaf pan, pressing into corners so that no air pockets remain.

☐ Bake in 350°F (180°C) oven for 50 to 60 minutes or until evenly browned and cake tester inserted in centre comes out clean.

☐ Let cool in pan for 10 minutes; remove to wire rack to cool completely.

Makes 1 loaf, 14 slices.

Calories per slice: 260
Grams fat per slice: 10.5
Grams fibre per slice: 4

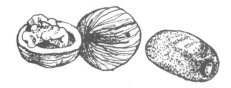

PEANUTTY COOKIES

Preparation time: 20 minutes
Baking time: 8 minutes

*T*hese cookies keep well if stored in a tightly covered container.

1/2 cup	shortening	125 mL
1-1/4 cups	packed brown sugar	300 mL
1	egg	1
3/4 cup	whole wheat flour	175 mL
1/2 cup	all-purpose flour	125 mL
3/4 tsp	baking soda	4 mL
1/2 tsp	baking powder	2 mL
1/2 tsp	salt	2 mL
1/4 cup	milk	50 mL
1-1/2 cups	bran flakes	375 mL
1 cup	unsalted peanuts	250 mL

☐ In bowl, cream together shortening and sugar until light and fluffy. Add egg and beat well.

☐ Mix together whole wheat and all-purpose flours, baking soda, baking powder and salt; stir into creamed mixture alternately with milk, mixing well after each addition. Stir in bran flakes. Chop 1/2 cup (125 mL) of the peanuts and blend into batter.

☐ Drop teaspoonfuls of batter onto greased baking sheets. Top each with 3 or 4 of the remaining peanuts. Bake in 375°F (190°C) oven for about 8 minutes or until golden brown. Let cool on pans for 2 minutes; transfer cookies to wire racks to cool completely.

Makes about 4 dozen cookies.

Calories per cookie: 74
Grams fat per cookie: 3.7
Grams fibre per cookie: 0.6

BANANA COCONUT BREAD

Preparation time: 20 minutes
Baking time: 50 to 60 minutes

*T*his popular lunch box favorite is made with a reduced amount of butter.

2 cups	**all-purpose flour**	500 mL
1 tsp	**baking powder**	5 mL
1 tsp	**baking soda**	5 mL
1/4 tsp	**salt**	1 mL
1 tbsp	**butter**	15 mL
3/4 cup	**granulated sugar**	175 mL
1 cup	**mashed bananas (about 2 large)**	250 mL
2	**eggs, beaten**	2
1/2 cup	**soured milk**	125 mL
1 cup	**shredded coconut**	250 mL

To sour milk for Banana Coconut Bread: Place 1 tsp (5 mL) lemon juice or vinegar in a measuring cup. Add milk to the 1/2 cup (125 mL) level. Let stand for 10 minutes, then stir.

☐ Mix together flour, baking powder, baking soda and salt; set aside.

☐ In large mixing bowl, cream together butter and sugar. Beat in bananas; add eggs and beat well. Alternately add dry ingredients and soured milk, stirring well after each addition. Add coconut; stir to blend.

☐ Pour batter into greased 9- x 5-inch (2 L) loaf pan. Bake in 350°F (180°C) oven for 50 to 60 minutes or until cake tester inserted in centre comes out clean. Let cool for 10 minutes in pan; remove to wire rack to cool completely.

Makes 1 loaf, or 12 slices.

Calories per slice: 207
Grams fat per slice: 5
Grams fibre per slice: 3.4

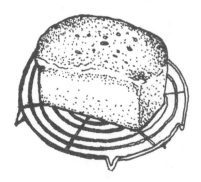

ZUCCHINI WHEAT GERM BREAD

Preparation time: 20 minutes
Baking time: 50 minutes

*T*his moist, not-too-sweet quick bread stores well for several days when wrapped tightly in plastic wrap or foil.

1 cup	shredded unpeeled zucchini	250 mL
2/3 cup	natural bran	150 mL
1 cup	lightly packed brown sugar	250 mL
1/2 cup	vegetable oil	125 mL
2	eggs	2
1/2 tsp	vanilla	2 mL
3/4 cup	whole wheat flour	175 mL
1/2 cup	all-purpose flour	125 mL
1/3 cup	wheat germ	75 mL
1 tsp	baking soda	5 mL
1/2 tsp	salt	2 mL
1/4 tsp	baking powder	1 mL
1/2 cup	chopped toasted almonds	125 mL

If you like a sweeter bread, add a lemon glaze to Zucchini Wheat Germ Bread just before removal from the pan. With a cake tester or skewer, poke holes all over top of loaf. Heat together 1/3 cup (75 mL) icing sugar and 1/4 cup (50 mL) lemon juice just until sugar melts and glaze is hot. Pour slowly over surface of loaf. Let stand for 10 minutes. Remove from pan and let cool before slicing.

☐ Toss together zucchini and bran; set aside. In large bowl and using electric mixer, beat together sugar, oil, eggs and vanilla for 3 to 4 minutes or until thick and foamy; stir in zucchini mixture.

☐ Mix together whole wheat and all-purpose flours, wheat germ, baking soda, salt and baking powder; stir in almonds. Add to zucchini mixture, stirring just until blended.

☐ Pour into greased 9- x 5-inch (2 L) loaf pan. Bake in 350°F (180°C) oven for 50 minutes or until well browned and cake tester inserted in centre comes out clean. Let cool thoroughly.

Makes 18 slices.

Calories per slice: 171
Grams fat per slice: 8.8
Grams fibre per slice: 2.3

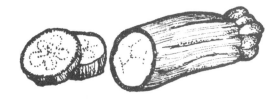

Notes

over: *Mustard Pork with Prunes (page 125), Potato Nests and Peas and Olives (page 128) and glazed beets.*

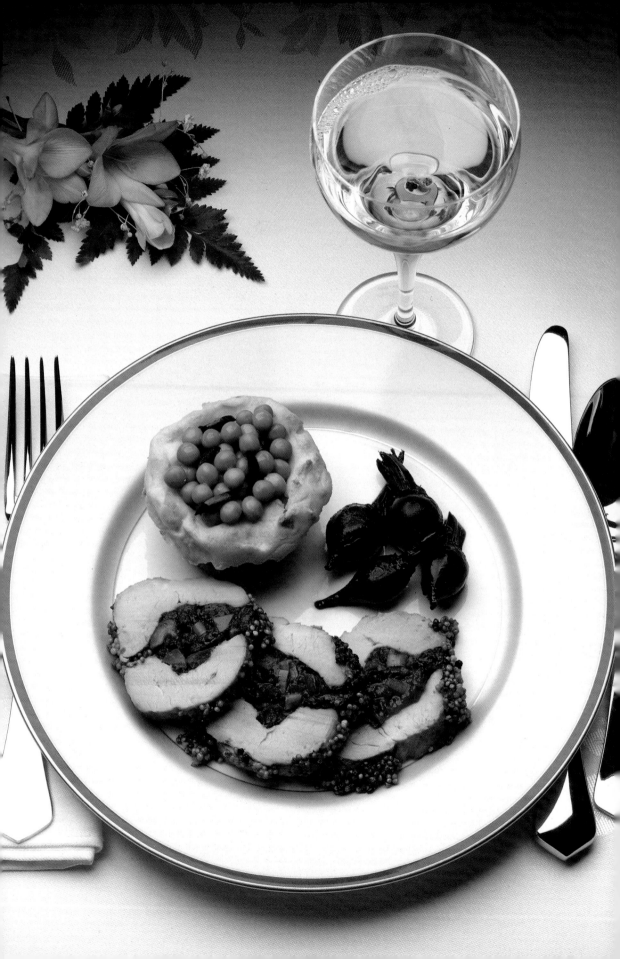

FIG BARS

Preparation time: 20 minutes
Baking time: 45 minutes

You can easily cut figs with floured kitchen shears. Be sure to remove any very coarse stem ends.

2 cups	**chopped figs**	500 mL
1/4 cup	**orange juice**	50 mL
1/4 cup	**butter**	50 mL
1 cup	**granulated sugar**	250 mL
1 tsp	**vanilla**	5 mL
2	**eggs**	2
1/2 cup	**all-purpose flour**	125 mL
1/2 cup	**whole wheat flour**	125 mL
2 tsp	**baking powder**	10 mL
1/4 tsp	**salt**	1 mL
3/4 cup	**chopped walnuts**	175 mL
1 tbsp	**icing sugar**	15 mL

☐ In saucepan, combine figs and orange juice; bring to boil. Reduce heat, cover and simmer for 4 to 5 minutes or until figs are slightly softened. Drain well. Let cool to lukewarm.

☐ In bowl, beat together butter, sugar, vanilla and eggs. Stir together all-purpose and whole wheat flours, baking powder and salt. Add to egg mixture; mix thoroughly. Stir in figs and nuts.

☐ Spread in greased 9-inch (2.5 L) square cake pan. Bake in 350°F (180°C) oven for 40 to 45 minutes or until lightly browned and firm to the touch. Dust with icing sugar while warm. Let cool and cut into 20 bars.

Makes 20 bars.

Calories per bar: 161
Grams fat per bar: 5.3
Grams fibre per bar: 4.1

PEANUT BUTTER COOKIES

Preparation time: 15 minutes
Baking time: 10 to 12 minutes

*P*opular with both young and old, these cookies have the added bonus of fibre.

1/2 cup	**butter**	125 mL
1/2 cup	**crunchy peanut butter**	125 mL
1/2 cup	**granulated sugar**	125 mL
1/2 cup	**lightly packed brown sugar**	125 mL
1	**egg**	1
1-1/4 cups	**whole wheat flour**	300 mL
1/2 tsp	**baking soda**	2 mL
1/2 tsp	**baking powder**	2 mL

For sparkling tops on Peanut Butter Cookies, dip fork into granulated sugar before flattening the cookies.

☐ In bowl, cream together butter, peanut butter, granulated and brown sugars and egg. Stir together flour, baking soda and baking powder; add to creamed mixture and beat until well blended. If dough is too soft to roll into small balls, chill for 30 minutes.

☐ Roll dough into 1-inch (2.5 cm) balls and place on ungreased baking sheet; flatten with floured fork. Bake in 375°F (190°C) oven for 10 to 12 minutes or until evenly browned.

Makes about 3 dozen cookies.

Calories per cookie: 79
Grams fat per cookie: 4.4
Grams fibre per cookie: 0.7

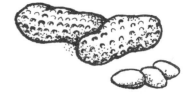

GOOD-FOR-YOU GINGERBREAD

Preparation time: 15 minutes
Baking time: 30 to 35 minutes

*T*his spicy gingerbread is fabulous served warm with either Nutmeg Sauce (page 161) or Tangy Orange Sauce (page 156). Or let the cake cool and dust it lightly with icing sugar. Two kinds of molasses are available in baking sections of supermarkets: fancy and dark. Fancy is the most widely used, but if you like a strong molasses flavor, use the dark.

1/3 cup	shortening	75 mL
1/3 cup	packed brown sugar	75 mL
2	eggs	2
3/4 cup	molasses	175 mL
3/4 cup	boiling water	175 mL
3/4 cup	100% Bran or All-Bran cereal	175 mL
2 cups	all-purpose flour	500 mL
2 tsp	cinnamon	10 mL
1 tsp	baking powder	5 mL
1 tsp	baking soda	5 mL
1 tsp	ground ginger	5 mL
1/4 tsp	salt	1 mL

Instead of serving Good-for-You Gingerbread hot with sauce for dessert, let it cool, then make a pretty pattern on top with icing sugar just before serving. Place a paper doily (or your own cut-out paper pattern) on top of the cake. Sprinkle icing sugar generously over top. Carefully remove doily and white sugar pattern will remain.

☐ In large bowl, cream together shortening and sugar until light. Add eggs and beat well; blend in molasses. Pour boiling water over bran cereal; add to creamed mixture.

☐ Stir together flour, cinnamon, baking powder, baking soda, ginger and salt; add to creamed mixture, stirring to mix completely. Pour into greased 9-inch (2.5 L) square cake pan.

☐ Bake in 350°F (180°C) oven for 30 to 35 minutes or until cake tester inserted in centre comes out clean. Cut into squares to serve.

Makes 9 servings.

Calories per serving: 285
Grams fat per serving: 8.8
Grams fibre per serving: 2.4

Excellent source of: Iron
Good source of: Calcium, thiamine and niacin

TANGY ORANGE SAUCE

Preparation time: 5 minutes
Cooking time: 15 minutes

Serve this smooth creamy sauce hot or cold with Good-For-You Gingerbread on page 155.

1/3 cup	**granulated sugar**	75 mL
2 tbsp	**cornstarch**	25 mL
1/4 tsp	**salt**	1 mL
2/3 cup	**buttermilk**	150 mL
1-1/3 cups	**orange juice**	325 mL
1	**egg, lightly beaten**	1
2 tsp	**butter**	10 mL

☐ In heavy saucepan, blend sugar, cornstarch and salt. Add buttermilk and stir to blend well. Gradually stir in orange juice.

☐ Cook over medium-high heat, stirring constantly, until mixture thickens and comes to boil. Stir some of the hot sauce into beaten egg, stirring constantly; return to remaining sauce in pan. Cook, stirring, over low heat for 2 minutes. Remove from heat and blend in butter. Serve hot or cold.

Makes 2 cups (500 mL) sauce, 1/4 cup (50 mL) per serving.

Calories per serving: 72
Grams fat per serving: 1.9

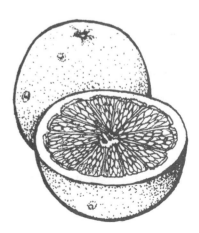

CHOCOLATE DATE CAKE

Preparation time: 20 minutes
Baking time: 35 minutes

*T*he unusual combination of dates and chocolate produces a cake with the wonderful texture of brownies.

1 cup	**chopped dates**	250 mL
1 tsp	**baking soda**	5 mL
1 cup	**boiling water**	250 mL
2/3 cup	**butter**	150 mL
3/4 cup	**granulated sugar**	175 mL
1	**egg**	1
1/2 tsp	**vanilla**	2 mL
3/4 cup	**whole wheat flour**	175 mL
1/2 cup	**all-purpose flour**	125 mL
1/2 cup	**unsweetened cocoa powder**	125 mL
1/2 tsp	**cinnamon**	2 mL
1/4 tsp	**allspice**	1 mL
1/4 tsp	**salt**	1 mL
1 cup	**chopped walnuts**	250 mL

☐ In small bowl, mix together dates and baking soda. Pour boiling water over and stir; set aside to let cool.

☐ In bowl, cream together butter and sugar until light and fluffy. Add egg and vanilla; beat well. Stir together whole wheat and all-purpose flours, cocoa, cinnamon, allspice and salt; stir into creamed mixture until completely blended. Add cooled date mixture; stir in nuts.

☐ Spread batter in well-greased 9-inch (2.5 L) square cake pan.

☐ Bake in 350°F (180°C) oven for 35 minutes or until cake tester inserted in centre comes out clean. Let cool and cut into 20 squares.

Makes 20 squares.

Calories per square: 205
Grams fat per square: 11.5
Grams fibre per square: 2

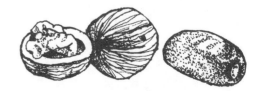

Notes

Desserts

Fresh fruits, especially ones listed as fibre-rich in the chart on page 5, make a great finale to a meal. But occasionally a special dessert is a pleasant change. Knowing a dessert is a good source of fibre somehow makes up for the added calories!

Choose a light dessert such as Raspberry Yogurt Mould or a warm and comforting Plum Kuchen or Apple Crisp Pie with a whole wheat crust, depending on the rest of the menu.

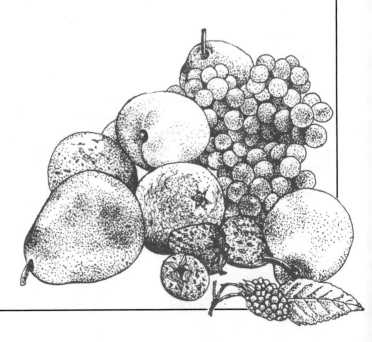

STEAMED APPLE DATE PUDDING

Preparation time: 15 minutes
Cooking time: 2 hours

Not quite as sweet as the traditional fruit pudding, serve this wintertime dessert with Nutmeg Sauce on page 159.

1	egg	1
1/2 cup	maple syrup	125 mL
1/2 cup	milk	125 mL
1/4 cup	packed brown sugar	50 mL
1 cup	all-purpose flour	250 mL
1/2 cup	whole wheat flour	125 mL
1 tsp	salt	5 mL
1/2 tsp	baking soda	2 mL
1/2 tsp	cinnamon	2 mL
1/4 tsp	freshly grated nutmeg	1 mL
1-1/2 cups	chopped unpeeled apples	375 mL
1/2 cup	chopped dates	125 mL
1/4 cup	cold butter, cut in small pieces	50 mL

To freeze Steamed Apple Date Pudding, wrap it in foil, seal tightly and label. Freeze for up to 3 months. To reheat: Bake thawed pudding, still in foil, in 350°F (180°C) oven for 1 hour or until heated through.

☐ In large mixing bowl, beat egg. Add maple syrup, milk and sugar; beat well. Stir together all-purpose and whole wheat flours, salt, baking soda, cinnamon and nutmeg; add to egg mixture, beating well. Stir in apples, dates and butter pieces.

☐ Pour batter into greased 4-cup (1 L) pudding mould or heatproof bowl. Cover tightly with greased foil or parchment paper, tying with string to secure tightly.

☐ Place mould on rack (a small metal jar lid will do) in large saucepan. Add enough boiling water to come 2 inches (5 cm) up side of mould. Cover and steam in simmering water for 2 hours (1-1/2 hours if using ring mould), adding more water to maintain liquid level if necessary.

☐ Remove pudding from steamer. Uncover and let stand for 5 minutes. Invert onto serving plate.

Makes 8 servings.

Calories per serving: 269
Grams fat per serving: 7
Grams fibre per serving: 2.7

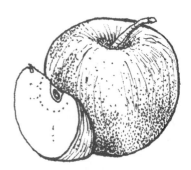

NUTMEG SAUCE

Cooking time: 10 minutes

*T*his smooth tasty sauce makes a perfect accompaniment for Steamed Apple Date Pudding on page 160).

1/4 cup	granulated sugar	50 mL
2 tbsp	all-purpose flour	25 mL
1/4 tsp	salt	1 mL
1-1/2 cups	milk	375 mL
1	egg, lightly beaten	1
2 tbsp	butter	25 mL
1/2 tsp	vanilla	2 mL
1/4 tsp	freshly grated nutmeg	1 mL

☐ In medium saucepan, mix together sugar, flour and salt; blend in milk. Cook over medium heat, stirring constantly, until mixture boils and is thickened and smooth.

☐ Stir a little of the hot sauce into beaten egg, stirring constantly; return to remaining sauce in pan. Cook, stirring, over low heat for 1 minute. Remove from heat and stir in butter, vanilla and nutmeg. Serve at once, or keep hot over simmering water.

Makes 1-1/2 cups (375 mL) sauce, enough for 8 servings.

Calories per serving: 83
Grams fat per serving: 4.3

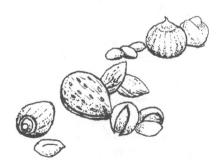

PINEAPPLE CHEESECAKE

Preparation time: 20 minutes
Baking time: 50 to 60 minutes

*A*t last, a cheesecake that is smooth and creamy but with a lot less fat than you would expect. A blender makes this cheesecake very smooth; a food processor may be used, but the result is slightly grainier.

Crust:

1 cup	graham wafer crumbs	250 mL
1/2 cup	ground almonds	125 mL
2 tbsp	packed brown sugar	25 mL
1/4 cup	butter, melted	50 mL

Filling:

2 cups	low-fat (2%) cottage cheese	500 mL
3	eggs	3
1/2 cup	lightly packed brown sugar	125 mL
1/2 cup	milk	125 mL
1/4 cup	all-purpose flour	50 mL
1 tsp	vanilla	5 mL
1/2 tsp	grated lemon rind	2 mL
1/4 tsp	lemon juice	1 mL

Topping:

1 cup	crushed pineapple (packed in juice), undrained	250 mL
1 tsp	cornstarch	5 mL
1/2 cup	dried apricots, chopped	125 mL
1 tbsp	apricot liqueur (optional)	15 mL

Garnish:

1/3 cup	toasted slivered almonds	75 mL

When berries are in season, top cheesecake with 2 cups (500 mL) fresh strawberries, raspberries, blueberries or blackberries. Make a glaze by combining 1/2 cup (125 mL) water, 1/2 cup (125 mL) granulated sugar, 3 tbsp (50 mL) lemon juice and 4 tsp (20 mL) cornstarch. Bring the mixture to a boil, stirring constantly. Remove from heat and let cool slightly. Spoon over berries on top of cheese-cake and refrigerate until set.

Crust:

☐ Combine crumbs, almonds, 2 tbsp (25 mL) brown sugar and melted butter. Press onto bottom and partway up side of 8-inch (2 L) springform pan. Bake in 350°F (180°C) oven for 7 minutes.

Filling:

☐ In blender or food processor, combine cottage cheese, eggs, 1/2 cup (125 mL) brown sugar, milk, flour, vanilla, and lemon rind and juice; whirl or process until smooth. Pour into prepared crust.

☐ Bake in 350°F (180°C) oven for 50 to 60 minutes or
until set. Immediately run knife around edge of pan to
release cheesecake, but do not remove side until completely
cool. Refrigerate until chilled.

Topping:
☐ In small heavy saucepan, combine pineapple with
cornstarch; stir in apricots. Cook over medium heat,
stirring constantly, for about 5 minutes or until mixture
boils, is thickened and clear. Let cool slightly; blend in
liqueur (if using). Spoon over chilled cheesecake.
Refrigerate until serving time. Garnish with nuts.

Makes 10 servings.

Calories per serving: 293   Good source of: Phosphorus
Grams fat per serving: 13.9
Grams fibre per serving: 2.9

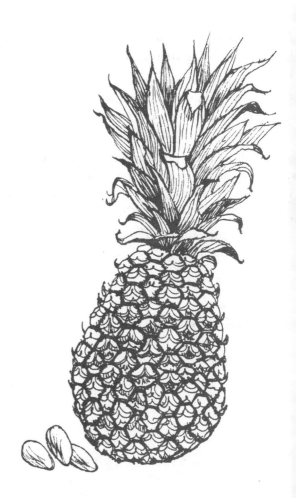

RASPBERRY YOGURT MOULD

Preparation time: 50 minutes
Chilling time: 4 hours

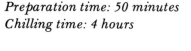

*T*his is a refreshing dessert to serve to family or friends. If sweetened raspberries are unavailable, mix 1/2 cup (125 mL) granulated sugar with either 3 cups (750 mL) frozen unsweetened raspberries (thawed) or 3 cups (750 mL) fresh berries.

1	package (425 g) sweetened frozen raspberries, thawed	1
2	envelopes unflavored gelatin	2
1/2 cup	orange juice	125 mL
1 cup	plain yogurt	250 mL
1 tsp	grated orange rind	5 mL
2	egg whites	2
2 tbsp	granulated sugar	25 mL

☐ Reserve a few raspberries for garnish. In blender or food processor, purée remaining raspberries; transfer to bowl.

☐ In saucepan, soften gelatin in orange juice; cook over low heat until gelatin has dissolved. Stir into raspberry purée and mix well. Add yogurt and orange rind; blend well. Chill until thick but not set, about 30 minutes.

☐ In bowl, beat egg whites until soft peaks form. Gradually beat in sugar; beat until stiff and glossy. Fold whites into raspberry mixture. Pour into rinsed 6-cup (1.5 L) mould. Chill until firm, about 4 hours.

☐ Unmould onto serving plate and garnish with reserved raspberries.

Makes 6 servings.

Calories per serving: 136
Grams fat per serving: 0.7
Grams fibre per serving: 7

Excellent source of: Vitamin C

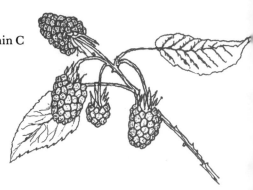

MERINGUE-TOPPED GRAPEFRUIT HALVES

Preparation time: 15 minutes
Baking time: 5 to 8 minutes

*I*f fresh cranberries are unavailable, use fresh sliced strawberries or drained crushed pineapple. Chopped walnuts or pecans can be substituted for Brazil nuts.

2	**grapefruit**	2
1/2 cup	**fresh cranberries, chopped**	125 mL
1/3 cup	**sliced Brazil nuts**	75 mL
1 tbsp	**liquid honey**	15 mL
1/4 tsp	**cinnamon**	1 mL
2	**egg whites**	2
1/8 tsp	**cream of tartar**	0.5 mL
2 tbsp	**packed brown sugar**	25 mL
8	**fresh strawberries**	8
	Mint leaves	

☐ Cut grapefruit in half. Remove sections to small bowl, discarding white membrane separating sections.

☐ Add cranberries to bowl along with nuts, honey and cinnamon; mix well. Spoon into 4 grapefruit shells and place in baking dish.

☐ Beat egg whites with cream of tartar until soft peaks form. Gradually beat in sugar until whites hold stiff peaks. Spoon onto grapefruit, spreading meringue to edges to seal in fruit. Bake in 400°F (200°C) oven for 5 to 8 minutes or until evenly browned. Garnish with strawberries and mint leaves.

Makes 4 servings.

Calories per serving: 153
Grams fat per serving: 7.5
Grams fibre per serving: 2.2

Excellent source of: Vitamin C

15-MINUTE MICROWAVE GINGER PEAR COBBLER

Preparation time: 15 minutes
Cooking time: 6 or 7 minutes
(Microwave)

*F*irm and ripe Bosc pears, available in the fall and winter, bake well. In season, Bartlett pears are a good alternative. This dessert is delicious with Nutmeg Sauce, page 161.

Fruit Layer:

5	**pears**	5
1/2 cup	**packed brown sugar**	125 mL
2 tsp	**cornstarch**	10 mL
1 tbsp	**lemon juice**	15 mL

Gingerbread:

1	**egg**	1
1/2 cup	**soured milk**	125 mL
1/4 cup	**light molasses**	50 mL
2 tbsp	**vegetable oil**	25 mL
1/2 cup	**whole wheat flour**	125 mL
1/2 cup	**all-purpose flour**	125 mL
1/4 cup	**packed brown sugar**	50 mL
1/2 tsp	**baking soda**	2 mL
1/2 tsp	**ground ginger**	2 mL
1/4 tsp	**ground nutmeg**	1 mL
1/4 tsp	**salt**	1 mL
1/4 tsp	**baking powder**	1 mL

To sour milk for 15-minute Microwave Ginger Pear Cobbler: Place 1 tsp (5 mL) lemon juice or vinegar in a measuring cup. Add milk to the 1/2 cup (125 mL) level. Let stand for 10 minutes, then stir.

Fruit Layer:

☐ Peel, core and slice pears. Blend together brown sugar and cornstarch; mix with pears along with lemon juice. Spoon into greased 10-inch (25 cm) microwave-safe ring mould dish. Microwave at High (100% power) for 4 minutes or until pears are just tender, stirring after 2 minutes.

Gingerbread:

☐ In mixing bowl, beat together egg, soured milk, molasses and oil. Stir together whole wheat and all-purpose flours, brown sugar, baking soda, ginger, nutmeg, salt and baking powder. Add to liquid ingredients; beat until smooth.

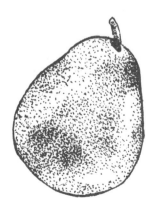

☐ Pour batter over pear mixture. Microwave at High (100% power), uncovered, for 6 to 7 minutes or until cake tester inserted near centre comes out clean. (If necessary, rotate dish twice during cooking.) Serve warm or cold.

Makes 6 servings.

Calories per serving: 355
Grams fat per serving: 6.6
Grams fibre per serving: 3.7

Good source of: Iron

BANANAS WITH MANGO YOGURT SAUCE

Preparation time: 10 minutes

This simple but refreshing dessert is quick and easy to make. The tart yogurt sweetened with brown sugar complements the exotic taste of mango.

1	mango, peeled and chopped	1
1 cup	plain yogurt	250 mL
1/2 cup	packed brown sugar	125 mL
1/2 cup	toasted slivered almonds	125 mL
3	large bananas	3

☐ In blender or food processor, purée mango, yogurt and brown sugar. Reserve 2 tbsp (25 mL) almonds for garnish; stir remaining almonds into mango mixture.

☐ At serving time, slice bananas into large bowl. Spoon mango sauce over top; sprinkle with reserved almonds.

Makes 6 servings.

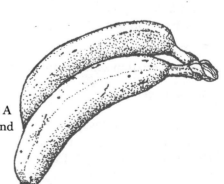

Calories per serving: 229
Grams fat per serving: 6.9
Grams fibre per serving: 3.8

Excellent source of: Vitamin A
Good source of: Vitamin C and
    riboflavin

PLUM GOOD KUCHEN

Preparation time: 15 minutes
Baking time: 40 minutes

*W*hen other fresh fruits are in season, you may want to vary this topping. Substitute sliced unpeeled nectarines, sliced peeled peaches or sliced peeled apples for the plums. This dessert is wonderful served warm and topped with a dollop of Mock Sour Cream, page 80, or plain yogurt.

Topping:

2 cups	**halved pitted prune plums (about 18)**	500 mL
2 tbsp	**packed brown sugar**	25 mL
1 tsp	**cinnamon**	5 mL
1 tsp	**grated lemon rind**	5 mL

Cake:

1/2 cup	**all-purpose flour**	125 mL
1/2 cup	**whole wheat flour**	125 mL
1/2 cup	**granulated sugar**	125 mL
1/2 tsp	**baking powder**	2 mL
1/4 tsp	**baking soda**	1 mL
1/4 tsp	**salt**	1 mL
1	**egg**	1
1/3 cup	**vegetable oil**	75 mL
1 tbsp	**lemon juice**	15 mL
1/2 tsp	**vanilla**	2 mL

You can make Plum Good Kuchen in an 8- or 9-inch (1.2 L or 1.5 L) round cake pan, but increase the baking time by 10 to 15 minutes or until cake tester inserted in centre comes out clean.

Topping:

☐ In bowl, toss together plums, brown sugar, cinnamon and lemon rind; set aside.

Cake:

☐ In mixing bowl, blend all-purpose and whole wheat flours, sugar, baking powder, baking soda and salt. Beat together egg, oil, lemon juice and vanilla; blend into dry ingredients. Spread batter in greased 9-inch (1.5 L) round cake pan; top with plum mixture.

☐ Bake in 350°F (180°C) oven for 40 minutes or until cake tester inserted in centre comes out clean.

Makes 6 servings.

Calories per serving: 294
Grams fat per serving: 13.1
Grams fibre per serving: 2.4

Notes

over: *Plum Good Kuchen (page 168).*

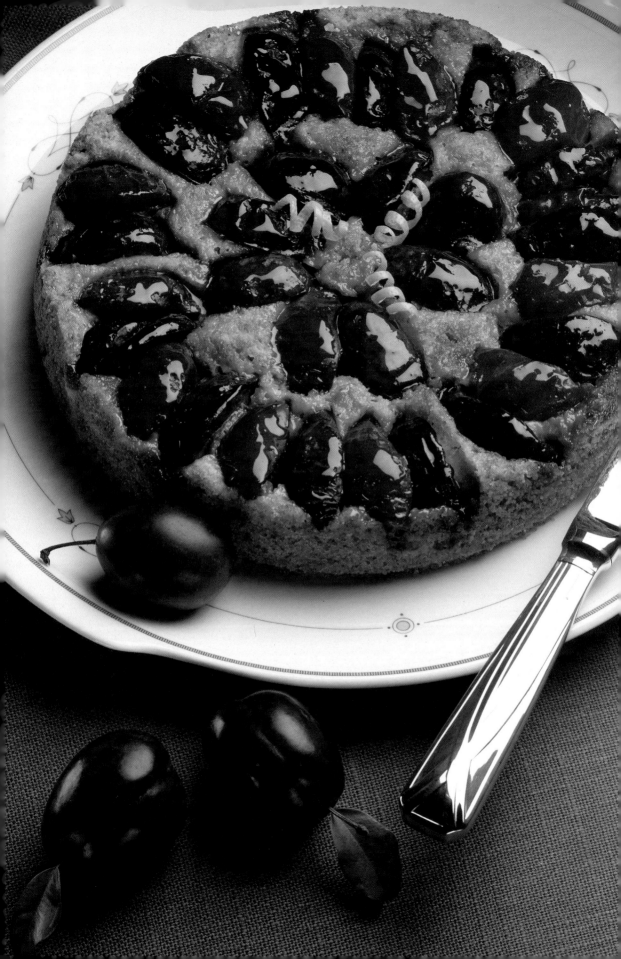

APPLE CRISP PIE

Preparation time: 20 minutes
Baking time: 40 minutes

*T*o please those who love apple crisp and those who love apple pie, serve this open-faced pie. The pastry can be used for other sweet or savory pies.

Pastry:

1/2 cup	100% Bran cereal	125 mL
1/2 cup	**whole wheat flour**	125 mL
1/4 cup	**all-purpose flour**	50 mL
1/2 tsp	**salt**	2 mL
1/4 cup	**shortening**	50 mL
1/4 cup	**(approx) ice-cold water**	60 mL

Filling:

2 tbsp	**apricot jam**	25 mL
2	**large apples, peeled and sliced**	2
1/3 cup	**granulated sugar**	75 mL
1/3 cup	**rolled oats**	75 mL
2 tbsp	**all-purpose flour**	25 mL
1/2 tsp	**cinnamon**	2 mL
1 tbsp	**butter**	15 mL

Pastry:

☐ In bowl, stir together cereal, whole wheat and all-purpose flours and salt.

☐ Using pastry blender or 2 knives, cut in shortening until in coarse crumbs. Sprinkle with cold water, 1 tbsp (15 mL) at a time, and toss with fork; form dough into ball. On floured surface, roll out pastry to fit 9-inch (25 cm) pie plate; flute edges. Chill for 30 minutes.

Filling:

☐ Spread apricot jam on pie crust; arrange apples over top.

☐ Mix together sugar, rolled oats, flour and cinnamon; cut in butter until mixture resembles crumbs. Sprinkle over apples. Bake in 425°F (220°C) oven for 10 minutes. Reduce heat to 375°F (190°C) and cover pie loosely with foil. Bake for 30 to 35 minutes longer or until lightly browned and filling is bubbly.

Makes 8 servings.
Calories per serving: 197
Grams fat per serving: 8.2
Grams fibre per serving: 3.2

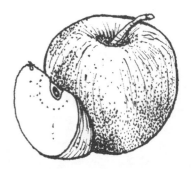

BAKED PINEAPPLE WITH COCONUT

Preparation time: 20 minutes
Baking time: 45 minutes

*I*n the summer, you can wrap this in heavy-duty foil and bake it on the barbecue. Turn back foil on top for second baking. Watch carefully because if your fire is very hot, this will not take as long to cook.

1	**large fresh pineapple**	1
1/2 cup	**orange marmalade**	125 mL
1/3 cup	**coarsely grated fresh coconut**	75 mL
1/3 cup	**chopped toasted almonds or macadamia nuts**	75 mL
1/4 cup	**slivered dried apricots**	50 mL
1 tbsp	**orange liqueur or orange juice concentrate**	15 mL

To toast almonds: Spread on baking sheet and bake in 350°F (180°C) oven for 5 minutes or until golden.

If you find it difficult to remove the pineapple from its shell for Baked Pineapple with Coconut, plan to serve the fruit mixture piled on individual scallop shells. Cover each with foil to bake. When done, serve each one garnished with shiny lemon leaves and a fresh flower.

☐ Using sharp knife, halve pineapple lengthwise, leaving crown intact. Remove fruit from both halves; cut into bite-size chunks, removing core.

☐ In large bowl, toss pineapple chunks with marmalade, coconut, nuts, apricots and liqueur. Place pineapple shells in shallow baking dish; spoon fruit mixture back into shells. Cover with foil, including crown.

☐ Bake in 350°F (180°C) oven for 30 minutes. Remove foil covering fruit mixture, leaving crown covered. Bake for 15 minutes longer or until top is lightly browned.

Makes 8 servings.

Calories per serving: 148   Good source of: Vitamin C
Grams fat per serving: 4.4
Grams fibre per serving: 2.7

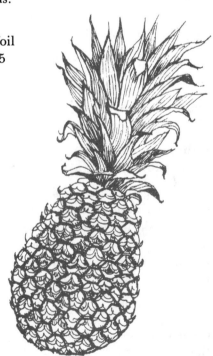

Miscellaneous

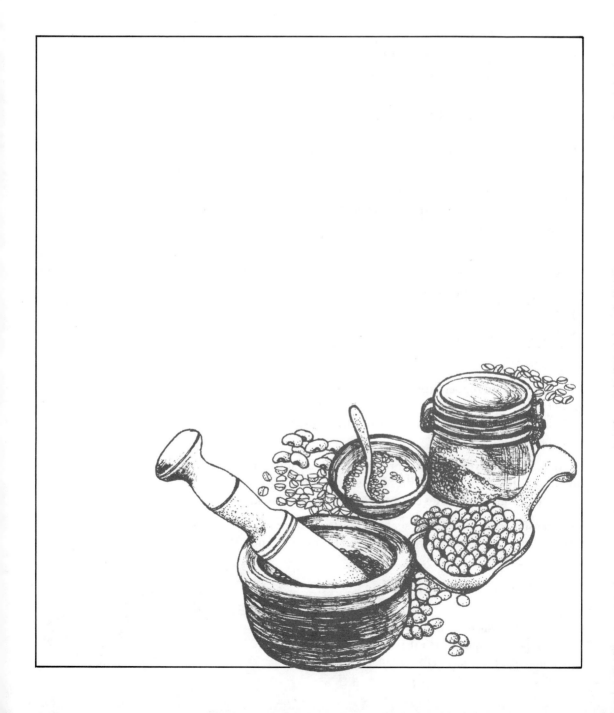

MANGO CHUTNEY

Preparation time: 15 minutes
Cooking time: 1-1/4 hours

*B*rimming with fruits and vegetables, this tasty chutney is a wonderful accompaniment to lamb, chicken, cold meats or curries. Use it to perk up Chutney Rice Salad, page 99, as well.

1 cup	packed brown sugar	250 mL
2/3 cup	cider vinegar	150 mL
1/3 cup	orange juice	75 mL
1 tbsp	grated orange rind	15 mL
2	mangoes, peeled, pitted and chopped	2
1	Granny Smith apple, peeled and diced	1
1	sweet red pepper, seeded and diced	1
1	medium onion, chopped	1
1 tbsp	finely chopped gingerroot	15 mL
1 tsp	dry mustard	5 mL
1/2 tsp	salt	2 mL
Dash	hot pepper sauce	Dash
5	whole cloves	5
1	cinnamon stick (2 inch/5 cm)	1
1/2 cup	golden raisins	125 mL

To sterilize jars: Place clean jars on baking sheet. Heat in 225°F (110°C) oven for 15 minutes. Place lids and screw bands in small saucepan and cover with boiling water. Boil for 5 minutes just before sealing jars.

☐ In heavy saucepan, stir together sugar, vinegar, orange juice and rind, mangoes, apple, red pepper, onion, gingerroot, mustard, salt and hot pepper sauce. Tie cloves and cinnamon stick in square of cheesecloth; add to saucepan.

☐ Bring to boil over high heat; reduce heat and simmer, uncovered, for 45 minutes. Add raisins; cook, stirring often, for about 30 minutes or until chutney is very thick.

☐ Transfer to sterilized jars; seal with lids and store in refrigerator. Or process in water bath for 10 minutes and store in cool dark dry place.

Makes about 2-1/2 cups (625 mL).

Calories per tablespoon (15 mL): 37
Grams fat per tablespoon (15 mL): 0.1
Grams fibre per tablespoon (15 mL): 0.4

GUIDELINES FOR COOKING BEANS, PEAS AND LENTILS

*T*he Food Advisory Division of Agriculture Canada has established cooking times for Canadian varieties of beans, peas and lentils. Although overall preparation time is still shorter for the quick-soak method, you will have to decide which method is more convenient since cooking times are longer for some beans soaked by the quick-soak method.

Most dried legumes (pulses) need to be soaked before cooking. Use either the quick-soak or the overnight-soak method. (Lentils and Split Peas do not require soaking. Suggested cooking time for lentils is 30 minutes; for split peas 50 minutes.)

QUICK-SOAK: Place peas or beans in a strainer and wash thoroughly. Discard any that are discolored. Transfer to large pot and cover with 3 to 4 times their volume of water. Bring to boil and boil for 2 minutes. Remove from heat, cover and let stand for 1 hour.

OVERNIGHT-SOAK: Place peas or beans in a strainer and wash thoroughly. Discard any that are discolored. Transfer to large pot and cover with 3 to 4 times their volume of water. Let soak overnight. (Refrigerate if your kitchen is warm.)

COOKING SOAKED BEANS (either method): Bring peas or beans to boil in soaking liquid. Cover and boil gently until beans are tender (see chart for times). Most beans double in volume when cooked.

COOKING TIMES FOR DRIED BEANS AND PEAS

TYPE	COOKING TIME FOR QUICK-SOAK METHOD	COOKING TIME FOR OVERNIGHT-SOAK METHOD
Romano (Cranberry) Beans	45 minutes	45 minutes
Great Northern Beans	1 hour	75 minutes
Kidney Beans — red	1 hour	1 hour
Kidney Beans — white	40 minutes	1 hour
Lima Beans — large	20 minutes	40 minutes
Lima Beans — small	35 minutes	35 minutes
Navy (pea) Beans	1-1/2 hours	50 minutes
Peas (whole) — yellow only	1 hour	40 minutes
Pinto Beans	45 minutes	45 minutes
Small Red Beans	50 minutes	40 minutes
Soy Beans	3-1/2 hours	4 hours

APPENDIX A
Eat a Variety of Foods from Each Group Every Day

Energy needs vary with age, sex and activity. Foods selected according to the guide can supply 1000-1400 calories. For additional energy, increase the number and size of servings from the various food groups or add other foods.

milk and milk products

Children up to 11 years	**2-3 servings**
Adolescents	**3-4 servings**
Pregnant and nursing women	**3-4 servings**
Adults	**2 servings**

Skim, 2%, whole, buttermilk, reconstituted dry or evaporated milk may be used as a beverage or as the main ingredient in other foods. Cheese may also be chosen.

Examples of one serving
250 mL (1 cup) milk, yoghurt or cottage cheese
45 g (1½ ounces) cheddar or process cheese

In addition, a supplement of vitamin D is recommended when milk is consumed which does not contain added vitamin D.

fruits and vegetables

4-5 servings

Include at least two vegetables.
Choose a variety of both vegetables and fruits—cooked, raw or their juices. Include yellow or green or green leafy vegetables.

Examples of one serving
125 mL (½ cup) vegetables or fruit
125 mL (½ cup) juice
1 medium potato, carrot, tomato, peach, apple, orange or banana.

bread and cereals

3-5 servings

whole grain or enriched. Whole grain products are recommended.

Examples of one serving
1 slice bread
125 to 250 mL (½-1 cup) cooked or ready-to-eat cereal
1 roll or muffin
125 to 200 mL (½-¾ cup) cooked rice, macaroni, spaghetti

meat and alternates

2 servings

Examples of one serving
60 to 90 g (2-3 ounces) cooked lean meat, poultry, liver or fish
60 mL (4 tablespoons) peanut butter
250 mL (1 cup) cooked dried peas, beans or lentils
80 to 250 mL (⅓-1 cup) nuts or seeds
60 g (2 ounces) cheddar, process or cottage cheese
2 eggs

Canada's Food Guide, Handbook. Ottawa: Health and Welfare Canada, 1977.

*A*PPENDIX B

Guidelines for Nutrient Ratings of Recipes:

Canada's "Food & Drug Regulations" (D.01.005 and D.02.004) sets out guidelines for rating nutrients in single servings of foods. Each food must provide specific amounts of each nutrient to be given a rating as either a good or an excellent source of that nutrient.

Nutrient	Good Source	Excellent Source
Vitamin A (IU)	600	1200
Thiamine (mg)	0.25	0.45
Riboflavin (mg)	0.40	0.75
Niacin (mg)	2.50	4.50
Vitamin C (mg)	7.5	15.0
Calcium (mg)	150	300
Phosphorus (mg)	150	300
Iron (mg)	2.0	4.0
Dietary fibre (g)	2.0–3.9	4.0 +

Dietary fibre was assessed following figures in the "Canadian Nutrient File".

INDEX:
Nutrition and Fibre

INDEX: *Fabulous Fibre Recipes*

An asterisk (*) indicates a recipe that is a good source of fibre but high in fat. Use occasionally.